THE ECONOMICS OF MEDICAL CARE

Edited by
M. M. Hauser

London. George Allen & Unwin Ltd
Ruskin House   Museum Street

ISBN 0 04 330213 0

Printed in Great Britain
in 10 point Times Roman
by Alden & Mowbray Ltd
at the Alden Press, Oxford

CONTENTS

FOREWORD

A. H. WILLIAMS
University of York

This volume is a product of tension, of confusion and of dissatisfaction. The tension is generated by the age-old gap between our aspirations for the provision of medical care and our capacity to satisfy them. The confusion exists over the respective roles and contributions of people with different skills in improving the performance of the system. The dissatisfaction arises because those most closely concerned with reviewing performance persistently feel that despite having so much effort, intelligence and goodwill at its disposal, the system still often responds in a disappointingly erratic and inefficient manner.

The role of economics in the medical care system is understandably a matter of some controversy. It generates a suspicion that ruthless, profit-seeking tycoons will be turned loose in a field in which it is rightly felt that humanitarian considerations should predominate. It is also seen as a potential threat to 'clinical freedom', to the notion that the practitioner's duty is to provide the best possible medical care for his patient, regardless of who the patient is and no matter what the cost. However, it is clearly unrealistic to suppose that the medical system does, or ever could, operate in this unconstrained way. 'Clinical freedom' is, and always has been, subject to the limitations imposed by lack of knowledge, lack of skill and lack of facilities. It still requires practitioners to exercise excruciatingly difficult judgements as to whether it is worthwhile their devoting further care and attention to a case where the return (in a purely therapeutic sense) is likely to be insignificant or even nil, and whether it would not be better to concentrate scarce time and skills instead upon cases where a greater payoff (in terms of improved health) is likely. Although not cast in terms of money these are, nevertheless, resource-allocation decisions, and are essentially what economics is about. Viewing them in this light, one speculates that it should be possible

9

to apply the corpus of economic reasoning, in order that we be not denied the insights which centuries of thought in that discipline have provided. But how could one do so?

Economists are not notorious for being shy, modest and retiring; nor are they oversensitive about demarcation lines between roles and disciplines; so it is not at all difficult to persuade economists that the health field presents resource-allocation problems on which economics (and hence economists) ought to have something useful and distinctive to say. Unfortunately, it is quite another matter to get any sizeable number of economists to commit themselves to working persistently and in depth in health problems, especially when there are so many other fields for the application of their skills which are better tilled and appear therefore to be more immediately productive. It is a pity that so few have so far responded to the challenges presented to economists by resource-allocation problems in the field of medical care, and it is to be hoped that as the importance and intellectual interest of these problems become more widely appreciated, this relative neglect will be made good.

One of the prime objectives of the conference out of which this volume grew was to bring together as many British economists as possible who had manifested a working interest in the economics of medical care, so that through the exchange of ideas and information each could derive stimulus and support, and future research effort could be more purposively directed and co-ordinated over the entire field. What we discovered very early on is that a great deal of the economics that is being done is being done by people who would not call themselves economists, but who have responded readily to the challenge and stepped into the shoes of the economists in order that the work be done, and not just left to go by default.

In publishing these papers, therefore, our twin purposes are to stimulate economists (and others willing to do economics!) to take more interest in the economic problems of medical care, and to indicate to non-economists the kind of role that economic reasoning can usefully and legitimately play in improving the performance of the medical care system.

It will be noted that the contributions range over a very wide field, and vary greatly in the conceptual apparatus they bring to bear and in the analytical techniques used. After Salter and Rudoe have laid out the resource-allocation problems facing those responsible for strategic decision-making in the National Health Service, Levitt formulates the general efficiency problem in a health context as typically seen by an economist. Cooper and Culyer then take one of the equity objectives of the NHS, that of geographical uniformity of provision, and, using very simple statistical techniques, investigate how far it has been achieved (and conclude that there is no evidence to suggest that such inequalities are diminishing). Crombie's model-building exercise is, in effect, a wide-ranging review of a great deal of work that has already been done on various bits of the system, with the objectives of pulling them all together into a more general framework of analysis and relating their conclusions to some of the present policy issues facing the health service.

After these general papers at a highly aggregated level, the next group tackles evaluative work on particular issues. Pole's study of mass radiography brings out very clearly the interplay of medical and economic considerations in assessing the worthwhileness of a medi-care activity, while Bevan's study on the divisions of certain responsibilities within a community health service highlights the need to focus evaluative effort on such organisational problems. In the final paper in this group Teeling-Smith offers some reflective comment on the lessons learned from the work of the Office of Health Economics since 1962, noting, in particular, that it has proved to be the exception rather than the rule that progress in medical care—and preventive medicine in particular—could normally be assumed to bring economic benefits of a kind conventionally measured in national income statistics.

The next group of papers concentrate on hospital planning. Beresford points out the shortcomings for management and planning purposes of cost data generated primarily for auditing accountability, but adds that quite simple reorganisation of that material can give some useful leads for improvements in efficiency. Luck shows how operational research techniques can be used in improving the managerial performance of the hospital, while Lavers sets up a framework for inferring from managerial behaviour what implicit relative valuation is being placed upon various medical treatments. Heasman pursues the associated theme of differences in consultant behaviour when faced with a similar array of cases, and comments on the need to provide acceptable incentives to promote professional acceptance of the desirability of change.

Two more general papers follow. The first, by Curnow, reviews the contribution that operational research techniques can make, returning once more to the need for a more clearly defined structure of authority within the health services and for the application of financial pressures to achieve beneficial changes. The second, by Sutcliffe, explores the implications of extending social accounting techniques into the medical care sector (public and private) as a means of elucidating the pattern of financial transactions and identifying the decision points in the allocation of funds.

Finally, in order that we do not get too introverted, there are three papers drawing our attention to what is going on in this field elsewhere, in Sweden (Spek), in France (Levy) and in the U.S.A. (Bowen and Jeffers). One cannot escape the overwhelming impression that despite cultural, social, political and organisational differences, we are all grappling with the same sort of difficulties and, although we can certainly profit from each other's experiences and results, none of us has yet found a satisfactory solution to our problems.

It would give a grossly misleading impression of the contents of this volume if I omitted mention of the contributions of the discussants of the various papers, which often go beyond comment on the paper to which they are related and offer, in addition, ideas and results emanating from their authors' own work, hence constituting valuable contributions in their own right. Finally, Hauser has written a synoptic account of our discussions, which, it will be seen, ranged not only over the subject matter of the papers themselves, but also ventured into important territory not covered directly in the written contributions (such as the role of consumer choice, the scope for the use of common yardsticks for performance between various activities, and the interplay of ethics and economics in the field of medicine). This makes Hauser's 'Summary of Main Points Raised in Discussion' something more than an addendum to the volume—it is worth reading for its own sake!

I hope that this cursory preview of the riches to be found within does not convey the impression that all the most interesting and important problems have now been dealt with, and all that is left for others to do is to dot the i's and cross the t's. The fact of the matter is that all the work reported here is of a pioneering nature. The authors would be the first to recognise the limitations of their respective contributions, and no one is yet in a position to assert that we know the right way to tackle any of the problems, still less that we have yet come up with any definitive answers. But when exploring unknown territory, patient probing on many points is frequently a rewarding strategy, and it is to be hoped that it proves so in the economics of medical care.

ACKNOWLEDGEMENTS

In 1970 a conference concerned with the Economics of Medical Care was held at the Institute of Social and Economic Research and the Department of Economics and Related Studies in the University of York. The papers in this volume are the outcome of this conference which it is hoped will be the first of a series of such meetings. The conference originated in an initiative of Professor J. Wiseman and was jointly sponsored by the University of York and the Department of Health and Social Security.

In addition to Dr M. M. Hauser who undertook organisational as well as general editorial responsibility, thanks are due to Mrs E. Heavens for her assistance with the administration and organisation of the conference papers and the conference itself, to Mr A. J. Cuyler for considerable editorial and other help, and to Mr R. J. Lavers. Miss S. Allen and Miss R. Shaftoe gave efficient secretarial help in the preparation of the manuscript.

Chapter I

OUTLINE OF PROBLEMS

PUBLIC EXPENDITURE AND THE HEALTH AND WELFARE SERVICES

H. C. SALTER

Department of Health and Social Security

This is not going to be a specialist contribution. I make no apology for that because the effect of our system of government is that, after all the specialists have given their advice, the crucial decisions are finally made by non-specialists—for example, by politicians. In fact, I see the basic intention of this symposium as being to discuss whether it would be worthwhile applying the specialist techniques of economic appraisal to help politicians and others, like me, who are not economists, to reach better decisions about the use of resources in the health and welfare field. By the end of the work we should see more clearly the extent to which economists and operational research workers may be able to help us to get an appropriate share of the national cake and, having got our share, whether they can help us to use it to the best advantage. I would add that although we are open to conversion to the use of more scientific methods of economic appraisal we do not envisage that they will ever become the sole indicators of how health and welfare decisions should be made. In the area in which we operate there are always likely to be moral, social and political factors to set alongside the economic ones, and in many cases decisions will have to be made which would be ruled out if judgements were made on economic grounds alone.

It might help to set the scene if I were to offer a few figures which show the order of magnitude of the problem we are dealing with and to write something about the processes which lead up to the decisions on what these figures should be.

In 1970/71 total public expenditure (including the nationalised industries and debt interest) is expected to be nearly £21,000 million or just over half the GNP. I propose to take this as given, since it is not our purpose to discuss what the level of total public expenditure should be or its relationship to the proper balance of the economy. Of this total, £1,920 million, or about 5% of the GNP, will be devoted to the health and welfare services. This compares with defence £2,211 million, housing £1,141 million, education £2,381 million and social security £3,738 million. The health and welfare figures are themselves further broken down as in the table below. This total is net of a

	£m.
Hospital capital	136
Hospital revenue	1,011
Family practitioner services	414
Community services capital	34
Community services revenue	232
Welfare foods	39
Miscellaneous	54
	1,920

number of charges. The gross amount which we shall be managing is £2,048 million.

In order to reach decisions on the amount of public expenditure there is every year an exercise called the Public Expenditure Survey which starts, at the lower levels of each spending department, with detailed forecasts of the costs of continuing existing policies over a five-year period. The first year is the year in which the exercise takes place and for which vote estimates have already been agreed, so, effectively the exercise is for four years. The forecasts build themselves up into national figures and, after discussions between the Treasury and the spending departments, are presented to ministers accompanied by a forecast of the state of the national economy over the same period. There will have been some adjustments to the individual figures during this process but no real weighing of the relative needs of each functional programme nor any judgement of priorities. Ministers are therefore likely to have before them forecasts of public expenditures which are in total more than the accompanying forecasts of what the national economy can bear. They will also have from each spending department an indication of the ways in which reductions in the forecasts would affect existing policies and probably of the directions in which the department thinks that more money should be allocated.

It is at this stage that one might expect that there should be some scientific judgement of priorities and of the merits of cutting one programme instead of another or even of increasing one programme at the expense of another. But at present there are no means of arriving at scientific assessments of priorities and decisions are taken mainly on political judgements, or on grounds of expediency or in relation to known public pressures. Among the social spenders it is only in education and to a small extent at the Home Office that a start has been made on analysis of objectives and on relating pro- grammes to them so that inputs can be allocated to objectives and related to the corresponding outputs. But changes are clearly com- ing. We have got so far as presenting to Parliament the new, annual White Paper on Public Expenditure. Although this is a considerable step forward Parliament may well feel that it needs more information to enable it to judge the relative merits of each functional programme. The Select Committee on Procedure has strongly advocated the development of output budgeting by government departments and envisages that this would ultimately be the basis for parliamentary discussion of priorities.

We are very conscious on the health and welfare side of the Department that in this new approach to judging priorities we may well lose in the struggle for a proper share of the national cake if we are not able to present our case more scientifically than we do now.

We think that the dangers for us are, firstly, that with new tech- niques of economic appraisal greater shares of public expenditure may go to those sections which can show clearly an economic return on investment and that an unconscious bias may develop toward favouring the economic rather than the social programmes. For example, a nationalised industry may be able to show a profit return on capital investment whereas at present we cannot demonstrate any comparable return from capital devoted to hospital building. Secondly, we fear that even within the social programmes health and welfare will suffer by comparison, for example, with education and roads because we cannot yet express our needs in mathematical terms nor show that better returns will come from increases in health and welfare expenditure as compared with increases in other outlets for public spending.

This presents us with a dilemma. We ought not to introduce new economic techniques just to be fashionable. We ought not to ask economists to use their scarce skills in producing economic measure- ments of the health and welfare services if the end result is likely to be highly artificial. But if we cannot find meaningful measurements of input and output we may be forced to go for the best we can devise, even though they may be somewhat artificial, simply in order to avoid being left behind in the struggle for our share of the national cake.

This then is the first question which needs an answer. It is to what extent can we use available skills in presenting a more effective case for health and welfare expenditure.

I do not intend at present to elaborate on the difficulties of producing economic measurements in the health and welfare field. No doubt they will all come out in discussion. But there are two particular points which I should like to make. The first is that public preferences and public pressures do, and should, play a part in decisions on the way public expenditure is shared out. In my view the health and welfare services are liable to lose out in this arena also. Most people can identify themselves with a campaign for better education, better roads, better housing or higher pensions, but there is a psychological barrier against identifying themselves with ill-health—perhaps even more so with prisons—and therefore the public pressures for improvements in these areas are not so great. Can any light be thrown on this and are there any ways of judging how the public range their preferences between programmes of public expenditure, even though there are no common measures of the value of these programmes?

The other point is whether there is any merit in arguing for a particular share of the GNP. Our share of the GNP has been compared one year with another and with other countries, but does this really get us anywhere and is it worthwhile making a closer study of what happens in other countries in order to get really relevant comparisons which might help our case?

The second broad area in which we feel that economists and operational research workers may be able to help us is in the judgements we have to make on what should be our priorities within the health and welfare services once our share of public expenditure has been allocated.

Probably the first thing to appreciate in considering this problem is that we have not a clean sheet to work on. There is already written over most of it the effects of the decisions of the past. It is near to impossible to alter these effects in the current year. It is difficult to do it for the next year—but at least next year there is a little extra to play with. In the third year there is a bit more scope for change. But it is not really until the fourth and fifth years that any significant effect can be made on the pattern of the main body of health and welfare expenditure. We are therefore operating on the margin although the margin does get appreciably bigger as we move further into the future. This makes it all the more important of course that we should start making more scientific decisions about priorities as soon as possible or we shall still be muddling along well into the 1970s.

At present the Department takes only very broad, long-term decisions on priorities—such as how much of our extra money should go to hospital capital, how much to hospital revenue and how much to the local authority services. Even these broad decisions are taken more as subjective assessments than as objective judgements of where the priority should lie. Very occasionally—as with our decision to set aside money to get a kidney-machine service started and our current decision to divert money to the care of the mentally subnormal —we make central decisions which have an impact on priorities. Very often we give advice to the hospital service about what should be done in particular fields. But we do not say what priority should be given to our various pieces of advice, and if each was followed the vote estimates would be greatly overspent. Over the great bulk of expenditure, therefore, decisions on priority are not made centrally. In default of that, they are taken locally—mainly by individual doctors and mainly quite unconsciously. The doctor who prescribes an expensive drug for a patient who will almost certainly die soon of cancer surely does not have it in his mind that this means that perhaps half a dozen people will continue to be away from work because of hernias. Even the central decisions I have mentioned—on kidney machines and care of the subnormal—were influenced in part by public pressure and by scandal. We did not judge—because we had no means of judging—whether these things really deserved on economic grounds the priority we were giving them. I must make it clear, however, that even if we had known the economic background we might still have made the same decisions for non-economic reasons. But at least we should have known what the economic cost of the decisions was and we might have been persuaded against them.

Of course, much of the reason for this unsystematic control of the NHS lies, historically, in the purposely loose rein with which we run it (apart from the overall financial control which on the hospital side is very tight) and in the complete clinical freedom given to the doctors who are the main initiators of spending. Perhaps we should discuss later what are the economic arguments for and against restricting that freedom.

Another of the reasons why we have never been very good at determining priorities is that we do not have available the information on which to make a judgement. It is really this question of getting the right information that we must start to look at soon if we are to make any progress in ordering our priorities more efficiently. In the hospital service, we know how much we spend on salaries and wages, on provisions, on fuel and so on. We know how much of these things is spent in maternity hospitals, in psychiatric hospitals, in acute hospitals and the rest. These are perfectly justifiable break-downs of expenditure for accounting purposes but they do not seem to tell us anything very meaningful when it comes to judging what we should increase and what we should do without. For example, the existing information does not tell us how much was spent on psychiatric treatment because the cost of this treatment in general hospitals is not separated out. But what is it that we do want to know? How should we be analysing the inputs into the hospital service? I cannot give an answer to these questions now. I can only ask other questions. Should we be analysing by types of illness? If so, can we think of some measurements of the value of the end result of treatment under each type? If we did that it would not be much good confining it to the hospital service. We should have to know what contribution the community services made in each case. This to me sounds a mammoth task, but perhaps we do not have to be very accurate and perhaps there are short cuts. Advice on this is wanted.

Some of this is straying very close to output budgeting and cost/benefit analysis, which will be discussed by others later, so I shall not develop my thoughts any further here except to make two points about cost/benefit studies. The first is that there is a perfectly reasonable argument that when a new development is looming over the horizon we ought to do a cost/benefit exercise before letting it get so far advanced that we cannot control it. But there is a danger in this—much the same as the one I referred to in the exercise of sharing out the national cake. It is that a development which can easily show an economic return may be preferred to another which, although intrinsically more valuable, might not be able to show an economic benefit so easily. The second point is that there is a tendency outside the Department to think that if expenditure of £x can be shown to have an economic return greater than £x then that is the end of the argument and the £x should be spent. This is unfortunately not so. We do not get credit, so to speak, for offsetting economic benefits and have to contain our expenditure within a predetermined total. Even though the benefits of spending £x may be obvious, we still may not be able to spend it—simply because we haven't got it.

One of our objectives in looking for an improved analysis of costs and expenditure and of outputs of the service is to enable us to assess what happens when we change one of the factors in the total situation. At present we lack the comprehensive picture which would enable us to know what happens if we make such a change. We do not know, for example, what would happen in the community services (or its cost) if substantial numbers of people were transferred from hospital to community care. We feel we ought to have the information which would enable us to do this sort of thing but we are not sure how to set about it and we wonder whether economists would be able to help us.

I have been concerned so far with determining priorities and following the most effective courses of action by using more scientific methods of economic appraisal or by operational research. But there is another area in which economists and operational research workers may be able to help us and this is in obtaining value for money. Since the annual increments for the health and welfare services are not likely to be very large it is probable that much of the new developments we should like to introduce will have to come from saving money in the main block of expenditure. If we can find out more about what the main body of expenditure now goes on, we shall be more able to decide whether anything can be discarded to make way for something new. But also we should be able to save some money simply by doing unavoidable things more efficiently. We already employ most of the normal aids such as O & M, work study, audit and the introduction of norms and standards. We are making a start on productivity schemes. But are there any other broader measures, such as the introduction of incentives and economic pressures, which we could adopt or any changes of policy which would enable us to get better value for money? Take the drug bill, for example, which we regard at present as very nearly uncontrollable except in terms of prices of drugs. Can economists help us to think of some completely new method of containing this cost? Or, conversely, can they help us to show that it should not be contained because of the benefits it causes in other parts of the health and welfare services?

I am very conscious of the fact that we need advice over a very wide field in which there are as yet many unknowns. I am fearful that because of this the immediate answer the economists and operational research workers would give is only that we must undertake a lot of research. Of course I accept that research will be necessary. But it takes so long. Ministers are in the dilemma that although many of their decisions do not take full effect for several years they in fact have to make some of them very soon after the problem becomes known. Very often decisions simply cannot wait for detailed and scientific study. Economists and operational research workers, if they are to help us, must therefore sometimes be prepared to provide argument and analysis without being able to suspend judgement while time-consuming research is going on. When long-term research is undertaken it must be clear that the right projects are being studied so that the answers when they come will still be to relevant questions and will not have been overtaken by events.

I shall finish by repeating that even when all the scientific techniques of economic appraisal are being used, the final decisions will sometimes be taken for reasons which an economist would regard as quite unrelated to the factors he thinks are important. Economists may find this discouraging and it may scare some of them away from working in the health and welfare field. I do not think it should, because it seems to me that there are large areas where economists will be able to exert an important influence. Moreover, if decisions do go against the logic of economic argument, it seems to me to be still right that the economic costs of making the decision should be established. This would be much better than, as now, making decisions without having full knowledge of what the costs will be.

ALLOCATION OF RESOURCES WITHIN THE HEALTH AND WELFARE SERVICES

W. RUDOE

Department of Health and Social Security

INTRODUCTION

There appear to be several peculiar difficulties in the application of economic concepts in the health field:

1. In general, the services are provided free. This means that the concept of demand, if taken to mean 'demand at a price', is not applicable. Substitution of 'need' leads one into deep and not very satisfactory waters.
2. We have no satisfactory measure of output and consequently no criteria for assessing productivity or determining allocation of resources according to the principle of equality at the margin.
3. A corollary of (1) is that health accounting leads to no 'profit' and with this another guideline to behaviour proves to be lacking.

How then can we get guidance from economists in a field where the usual economic criteria appear to be absent? An important field for research is an analysis of how the health services work at present. This covers not only detailed model-building of, for example, the functioning of a hospital on which a good deal of operational research is concentrating at present, but also a study of how decisions about the allocation of resources are made at present both at headquarters and regionally and locally. The Department is financing a good deal of health services research of a non-clinical kind relating to studies of the need for services, the use made of them and the way in which they are managed or organised. In many cases these studies are being conducted by multi-disciplinary teams and one question to which we would direct attention is the part which economists can play in such teams. The Department's view is that economic help is certainly required in some studies if only to crystallise some of the concepts.

Economists may be particularly helpful in the evaluation of experiments in alternative methods of providing care.

OBJECTIVES OF THE NATIONAL HEALTH SERVICE

Returning to the requirement of making 'the best use of resources' it can be seen immediately that this is quite vague since what do we mean in this context by 'best'? It might help us if we could define the objectives of the NHS and, moreover, define them in such a way as to give us guides to action and measures of what we are achieving. In the business world one assumes that the ultimate objective is to maximise profit in the provision of goods and services: *The Times* may choose to sell one product and the *News of the World* a somewhat different one, but philanthropy is not assumed to play a big part; firms which have chosen to sell something which is good but not at the same time profitable have foundered—or been bought by others who can use their assets more profitably. What then are the objectives of the NHS? The Act, says the Minister, has the duty of providing a comprehensive health service, but this is not explicit enough for our purpose. One could say that the objective is to maximise the health of the community as far as possible for a given expenditure of resources. This implies that we should seek to measure health, or at any rate the changes in health brought about by the NHS. There is a whole spectrum of activities from open-heart surgery, renal dialysis, etc. to varicose veins, hernias, septic fingers, etc. Choices have to be made—opening this special operating theatre may in effect delay the giving of less special treatment to somebody who, while less seriously ill, may be suffering considerable discomfort and be absent from work. Can we assume that the way such decisions are made now is about right? Traditionally, decisions about medical priorities are not usually reached by quantitative analysis. They tend to be reached by the pressure of public opinion or particular professional groups, the accident of a particular person in a particular spot, the development of medical technology, etc. A chain of events on which our medical colleagues might like to expand concerns renal disease. Here there has been progress from inevitable death in uraemia to intermittent dialysis, and from there to kidney transplants, while at the same time research is proceeding on the early detection of urinary infection and the prevention of kidney disease. The basic question seems to be: can we usefully manage to quantify in a field where human relations and compassion are so important?

PERFORMANCE AND EFFICIENCY

Taken overall, there is no measure of the output of the health service. The measurement of performance is of course linked with the definition of objectives: if you don't know what you are trying to do it becomes impossible to measure how well you are doing it. As a final end-product one can perhaps consider indices of mortality. However, the most striking changes, in the past at any rate, in mortality rates may have been due to improvements more in environmental health, water supply, etc. than in the operations of the health services as such. Moreover, now that infectious diseases are no longer so important, mortality rates are changing very slowly and are not good indicators of the performance with respect to chronic disease. Comprehensive measures of morbidity are at present lacking and it is clear that if use of services were taken as a measure, the continuous increase shown would be misleading. Leaving aside for the moment these general problems, we are nevertheless faced with the problem that if we are to compare alternative methods of providing medical care, or indeed to compare two institutions providing the same type of care, we need to be able to measure the outcome. At the moment, for instance, in the case of hospitals we can look at throughput per bed or cost per case. This is certainly some measure of output, but it does not seem to include any measure of the quality of the output. Perhaps as a first approximation it is good enough. But are we right to assume that we can treat the hospital in isolation and not consider what happens to the patient after discharge when he may need treatment in other parts of the NHS, or at home, or indeed may need to return to hospital again? In some areas the follow-up may be much more important than in others. We also need to think about what treatment may avoid the need for hospital admission. Furthermore, even if we could work out agreed measures of performance there would remain a substantial problem of putting into effect changes which would lead to improvement of performance. This is not to deny that such problems exist in industry too, but the organisation of the health service and the clinical freedom of the doctor do seem to lead to special difficulties. Quite a few measures of performance exist already but one is not sure how much regard is paid to them.

Again, in the business world, one has return on capital employed or income/assets ratios and these are diligently studied in the market and affect the firms concerned. Can we produce measures of significance in the health field and is it desirable that they should be closely followed? Could changes only be brought about by the pressure of example or could more positive steps be taken? It is no use working out measures of efficiency if they are going to be put aside as inappropriate for this service. This has proved to be one of the basic difficulties of operational research in health services so far.

OUTPUT BUDGETING

The previous paragraphs have talked about objectives and outcomes. Perhaps the specification of both has some way to go yet. But is there a way of categorising what the NHS is doing which will be meaningful and help us along this road? At the moment, broad financial figures are available on inputs, e.g. costs of hospitals can be broken down into the cost of labour and materials. We have figures of cost per case in hospitals of certain types. But only in the most approximate way do we have the costs of treating the conditions for which NHS exists, i.e. the money spent on bronchitis, heart disease, old people, young people, preventive medicine, etc. Is it worthwhile expending scarce resources in the Department on thinking out the appropriate categories and getting out the figures (which need not be 'accurate' but should be better than guesses)? Some say there would be no merit in this, since the incidence of disease produces patients in given proportions and they have to be treated. While accepting that there is something in this argument, I do not agree that the framework is as rigid as this. Patients in each category have to be treated—agreed—but with what degree of intensity and with which resources? Is this dependent entirely on the state of medical technology at the time? And what determines this? Is it solely the interest of the subject or the direction taken by medical education? What we want to know is whether we are spending the money now so as to maximise 'health' or whatever our objectives really are and what changes we need to make to do so. But even without this knowledge, we surely ought to know in output categories what we are spending our money on. Even without the precise setting out of objectives, the results might be sufficiently indicative of areas where close investigation was required, and would payoff in terms of better 'value for money'. Would the evaluation of costs of new procedures in advance, for example, affect our attitude toward them or would the pressures to which reference was made earlier prove irresistible? We recognise that the Office of Health Economics has carried out an approximate costing for broad categories of diagnosis. How significant is the undoubted error that there must be in these calculations? This will clearly depend on how one proposes to use the information, and here is a further problem: is the diagnostic classification the most useful or appropriate one to give us guidance on alternative courses of action?

SCREENING
We had thought that the evaluation of screening procedures by cost-benefit analysis was especially suitable for economic analysis, but in practice it has proved very difficult because a good deal of the information required does not seem to be available. It raises a complex of problems: medical knowledge of what to do according to the values of the parameters measured; the natural history of the disease in the presence and absence of treatment; the cost of finding a case needing treatment; the cost of treatment, particularly if this is applied at an earlier than clinical stage; the quantification of benefit. Work in this field will probably be justified although it still has a long way to go.

MANPOWER PLANNING
The NHS is labour-intensive and employs a wide range of people, from virtually unskilled porters and domestics to highly skilled professionals requiring long training. Errors in forecasting the need for doctors, for example, are not easily corrected. How to forecast this need is, however, still a subject of some controversy. One way of going about it is to consider the structure, e.g. taking hospital doctors, to evaluate the requirements allowing for progression to consultant status at a certain age and feeding in training needs, etc. The other way is to look at total need, using as a guide here the doctor/population quotient. This, however, is far from being a satisfactory indicator for forecasting when there is the possibility of using medical manpower in different ways from those employed at present. It becomes particularly difficult when the whole pattern of medical care is being rethought; one should be aware of the Green Paper on the reorganisation of the NHS and the parallel line of thought illustrated

by the 'best buy' and the 'community' hospital and the development of health centres. There are other complex problems, e.g. in the nursing field. One can attempt to determine minimum staffing ratios (nurses per patient) based on subjective assessment—or ratios which give a satisfactory standard of care—again subjective. Studies have shown wide variations, so that the demand is none too easy to quantify. Supply can to some extent be predicted, e.g. by looking at forecasts of the number of women aged 15–19, etc. coming forward in future years. Such women work in other industries too; does one assume, if total projected demand exceeds total projected supply, that all will go equally short? Will the NHS lose out in such a situation? What action needs to be taken? Are the demand projections right? What changes in the number of nurses will be required through changes in technology? The hospital is a very complex organisation indeed and one is constantly making assumptions that one can take an element out and study it in isolation. This may be so, but essentially one does this because of the difficulty of studying the total system. Operational research is making an attack on these problems, but economic expertise would clearly be valuable here too.

Chapter II

EFFICIENCY AND EQUALITY IN MEDICAL CARE PROVISION

PROBLEMS OF EFFICIENCY[1]

M. S. LEVITT
H.M. Treasury

INTRODUCTION

The formal economic properties of an efficient system of medical care are fairly easily established. It is in the translation of these ideal requirements into practice that the difficulties lie. This paper briefly outlines primarily for the benefit of the non-economist, the theoretical aspects of efficient medical care and considers the nature of the information and decision-taking systems needed to ensure the attainment of social priorities in the field of health at the lowest cost.

THE ECONOMIC PROPERTIES OF EFFICIENT MEDICAL CARE

The economic properties of efficiency in the production of medical services are no different from those in any other economic activity:

1. Each 'output' from the medical care system should be produced at the lowest cost; this involves the choice of the particular combination of inputs (e.g. drugs, nurses, doctors, etc.) which costs least per unit of output (e.g. patient treated).
2. The share of each particular activity within the medical service (e.g. maternity care, dental care) in the total resources available to the medical care, of each activity, must be consistent with society's relative priorities.
3. The share of medical care in total national resources must be consistent with societies relative preferences for medical care and alternative resource uses.
4. The availability of medical care to each individual must be in accordance with society's distributional objectives.

Before we can begin to translate these theoretical requirements into operational practices we need to decide how society makes its objectives known; we must know the cost of medical care and be

[1] The paper expresses the author's views, not those of his Department.

clear about what we mean by 'output' in the context of medical care.

SOCIAL OBJECTIVES

The notion of economic efficiency involves the consideration of costs and of objectives, but how does 'society' make its objectives known? One answer is that society's objectives in the field of health are those which individuals would reveal if the market mechanism were permitted to operate. Both the total resources to be devoted to medical care and the amount for particular medical services would, it is argued, conform to the objectives of society's individual consumers if they were free to decide for themselves how much to spend on medical care. It is alleged that when consumers are not faced by prices their demands are excessive and the supply, being dependent on competition for tax revenue, tends to be inadequate. Therefore, rather than have officials make decisions about allocation, individuals should be free to choose their consumption of medical care on the basis of prices which cover the costs of meeting their demands. To the extent that certain individuals are too poor to exercise much freedom of choice, their incomes should be supplemented. Insofar as individuals are unaware of the benefits from expenditure on medical care, publicity and improved education are required. There is said to be little chance of exploitation of patients since profit is not a dominant motive in private health services. Large emergency outlays can be insured against privately.

Against the above approach it can be argued that the conditions needed for optimal allocation via the price mechanism are not present. Competition between doctors and between hospitals is largely restricted. Equal knowledge on the part of consumers and producers is absent so that consumers need to rely upon medical opinion, with the result that doctors rather than consumers are really the decision-makers. Effects external to the individual are present, e.g. communicable diseases. Insofar as the profit motive is weak, much of the case for reliance upon the market mechanism collapses. In practice, means tests may be difficult to apply. The poor may postpone visits to doctors until ill health is serious. Those too poor to pay for hospital treatment or for private insurance may receive sub-standard facilities. It may become difficult to avoid costly or inessential treatment, e.g. gynaecologists where a midwife will do.

Insurance schemes sometimes bias the market in favour of hospitalisation, resulting in the under-provision of effective, cheaper alternatives. The upshot of this approach is the argument for a national health service, with the state judging society's objectives and priorities.

The first approach presented above seems to suggest that what is relevant to the utility functions of the relatively well-off, is the inability of the poor to purchase medical care should they choose to: all that is needed is an income supplement for the poor rather than public medical care. The second approach suggests that it is ill health *per se*, irrespective of income, that is relevant to our utility functions.

The choice between the two approaches is not only a choice between economic philosophies, it also involves judgement about the nature of the alternative outcomes; in particular it involves different estimates of the likely health standards of the poor under a market system. In practice, most medical care in the United Kingdom is provided publicly so that the setting of objectives and priorities is largely a matter for the state. However, as under a private system, doctors also enter into the system as being decision-makers in respect of forms of treatment, queuing priorities, technological innovations to be adopted, etc. The medical profession's role in decision-making is important and account should be taken of it in attempts to establish the determinants of public expenditure on medical care. The remainder of this paper is largely concerned with efficiency under present NHS arrangements.

THE COST OF MEDICAL CARE

The allocation of resources within the health service takes place under an overall budget constraint which sets the total cost of medical care. However this 'cost' has a number of dimensions depending on the relevant scope of the definition to be used and the time period to which it refers.

The total cost of public medical care at present, or in the past, is the opportunity cost of foregone alternatives. This is measured by comparing total public expenditure on medical care with gross domestic product, both at current factor cost. However, the cost to taxpayers is less than this, since one must deduct receipts from national health insurance payments and receipts from charges from total public expenditure. Thus in 1968/69, gross public expenditure on health and welfare of £1,892 million was reduced to £1,602 million after receipts.[2]

When one turns to the future costs of medical care, allowance has to be made for changes in relative prices. Let us assume a given population with given medical characteristics and a given state of medical knowledge. It does not follow that public expenditure (whether gross or net) will be a constant share of GDP at 'current prices' over time: 'This is because increases in productivity in the private sector will be reflected in increased output at constant prices, while increases in productivity in the public sector will be ignored except in cases where a given task is performed by fewer staff. Furthermore, rising productivity in the private sector will be accompanied by rising real earnings which tend to be matched by public sector real earnings.'[3]

In other words, the cost of public medical care will tend to rise relative to GDP and allowance has to be made for this.

The rise in relative costs is associated with the manpower element in current costs, measured at factor cost. For total current public expenditure this 'relative price effect' has been in the range $1\frac{1}{2}$ to 2%.[3] Medical care is more labour-intensive than the average public service and the relative price effect in respect of medical care is at the top end of the range, about 2%. Clearly when this is applied at compound rate over a number of years to a programme which is otherwise constant a significant addition has to be made, over 10% after five years, if we are interested in the share of medical care in total resources.

The increase in the public expenditure costs measured by including the relative price effect may understate the increase in the opportunity costs of medical care if Professor Kaldor's argument in his 1966 Inaugural Lecture is correct. Basically he argued that productivity growth depends upon the size of the manufacturing labour force. If one were to argue that the growth of the medical care labour force is in part at least at the expense of manufacturing then, if Kaldor is right, some productivity growth, i.e. additional income, is foregone. This loss will not show up in the statistics of GDP, nor will it show up in the relative price effect, which is related to actual, not potential,

[2] H.M. Treasury, *Public Expenditure 1968–69 to 1973–74*, Cmnd. 4234, Table 1.7 (H.M.S.O.).

[3] *Ibid.*, p. 78.

productivity growth. In the coming decade we will have a virtually static labour force but a growing dependent population. The medical care services will therefore be competing for a nearly constant labour supply so that, if correct, Kaldor's argument is important.

One reply to the argument of the last three paragraphs is that our accounting conventions ignore the value of improvements in the scope and quality of medical care output. However, before we can seriously consider trying to change our national accounting conventions we should be clear about what we mean by the 'output' of medical care, and about how we measure that output.

ALLOCATION WITHIN THE FIELD OF MEDICAL CARE

Efficient allocation within the total medical care programme involves the provision of each output at least cost, and the allocation between outputs in conformity with explicit choices. We need information about the nature and quantity of medical care output and about costs of achieving outputs through alternative methods, analysis of alternative allocations between outputs, and a system for making efficient choices on the basis of an evaluation of this information. The operation can be regarded as *an attempt to establish production functions* for given outputs (what is the maximum output, e.g. number of patients treated, suffering from a certain illness, which can be obtained by various alternative allocations of £x between the inputs, e.g. nurses, doctors, drugs?), *transformations between outputs* (if we reduce expenditure on type A patients by £y, assuming it was efficiently allocated, and raise expenditure on type B patients also efficiently allocated, how many fewer of A do we treat and how many more of B?) *with a view to allocating according to priorities* (do we want to reallocate £y from A to B?).

Before proceeding to decisions on how resources should be allocated, we need to know how resources are being allocated. We need to clarify our objectives so that we can be clear about our intended outputs. Medical objectives are those such as:

(a) training of manpower,
(b) control and prevention of disease,
(c) treatment of illness,
(d) care for the chronically sick and the aged, and
(e) research.

Within each broad objective, there will be narrower objectives, such as the training of specific types of medical manpower or the treatment of particular types of illness.

Allocation between outputs is multi-dimensional. It would be valuable to know not only allocation between medical categories such as those above, but also between age groups, economic groups, income groups, and regions. We can then establish multi-dimensional output groups, e.g. young disabled, chronically sick, aged poor, etc., with a view to reviewing allocations should our priorities warrant it. Further, this sort of disaggregation is needed in attempts to forecast the demands likely to be made upon the medical service in future. Some of the information needed for these purposes is already available from in-patient inquiries.

This information is essential for an evaluation of the distributional impact of medical care. An interesting recent publication by the U.S. Department of Health and Welfare summarises some of the relevant information for the U.S.A.[4] Differences in the standard of health and in the availability of medical care were found between regions and between the white and non-white populations. Considerable differences were also found between income groups: e.g. under half of the low-income children with chronic conditions or defects of hearing or vision receive treatment, although two-thirds of these disorders could be prevented or corrected if the appropriate health services were available. In this country the In-patient Enquiries provide information about patients grouped according to diagnostic, age and regional classifications. This information is useful for purposes of forecasting future demands on the health services except insofar as people in need of treatment do not come forward for it and so do not appear in the enquiries—which only, therefore, describe the 'tip of an iceberg'. Further, the information does not reveal the socio-economic impact to the health services.

We also need information, for any output group, of the production allocation—which also is multi-dimensional, e.g. between inputs (doctors, nurses, drugs, etc.) and between the location of treatment (in-patient, out-patient, at home). This information should be about current practices and alternatives, with a view to establishing the most efficient method, by techniques such as cost-effectiveness and

[4] U.S. Department of Health, Education and Welfare, *Towards a Social Report*, Washington, January 1969 (U.S. Government Printing Office).

by the establishment of production functions. In this country there is scope for comparative studies, building on the information provided in the hospital costing returns, with a view to explaining differences in hospital costs and efficiency.

Allocation also occurs over time. Time is of great importance in medical care, where long leads are present, e.g. in hospital building, medical manpower training. Our current decisions need to take account of prospective demands many years ahead. Also since our current decisions have expenditure consequences which may not be felt fully for several years it is important to establish priorities between the prospective demands in order to ensure that our future activities can be effectively carried out within the overall constraint upon resources likely to be felt in future.

OUTPUT

From the information described in the last four paragraphs we should obtain a multi-dimensional picture of how our resources are allocated between objectives and inputs, and of the consequences of alternative allocations. The point of the exercise is to arrive at a position in which one can specify an efficient allocation of resources: insofar as the 'efficient' allocation differs from practice, adjustments to our actual operations will be needed. The whole argument so far assumes that we can identify the output from the health services and that we can measure this output.

In the first place we need to distinguish the contribution of medical care to health as opposed to that of other influences, e.g. rising incomes. For medical care as a whole it is extremely difficult to devise output measures. Admittedly, overall indicators such as life expectancy at birth or infant mortality are available, but changes in the values of these indicators cannot be wholly associated with medical care. In the United States, despite a large increase in expenditure on medical care over the last decade, life expectancy has hardly improved. This does not mean that there are no possible improvements in the health of the U.S.A., since fifteen countries have a longer life expectancy than the U.S.A. The relationship between total medical care and overall health, as measured by life expectancy, is obscured by changes in living standards and conditions, which themselves have a complex relationship to health (improved diets and excessive consumption; more leisure but less exercise and more car accidents), and by changes in the characteristics of ill health (some diseases decline, others become more important). For purposes of resource allocation we are interested in marginal adjustments within the health service, so that ideally we need a common output measure for the whole service, e.g. the contribution to life expectancy. In practice we have to make do with output measures, such as the number of hospital beds constructed, doctors trained, patients 'discharged or dead'. Ideally we want to know the contribution of expenditure on hospital building and medical training to the nation's health; details of the number discharged do not tell us this, since we need to follow up the patients to see what becomes of them.

One overall measure which is suggested from time to time is the contribution to national income of medical care, as measured by the earnings of those whose working life is prolonged; this measure, however, conflicts with the objective of improving the health facilities available to low-income groups. For the time being, therefore, we must make do with a variety of measures, some nearer to ultimate measures of health than others.

PROGRAMME BUDGETING

The paper has outlined the requirements of an economically efficient system of medical care. Whatever precise administrative structure is chosen and whatever that structure might be called we cannot escape the requirements about objectives, priorities and information about alternative costs and outputs. The programme, planning, budgeting system which operates in the U.S.A. was specifically designed to meet these requirements. Prior to the introduction of a PPB system in 1967, health programmes were largely a collection of bids put up by various parts of the system to the Secretary, who provided no guidance about priorities. 'It was usually assumed that existing expenditures were an inviolate base, not requiring re-examination.'[5] Despite the long leads in health programmes, the planning horizon was only one year ahead. New proposals were not rigorously evaluated in relation to existing programmes. The overall programme review was largely concerned with the administrative feasibility of the expenditure and with the prospects for 'selling' it to Congress.

[5] R. N. Grosse, 'Problems of Resource Allocation in Health', Vol. 3 of: *The Analysis and Evaluation of Public Expenditures: The PPB System*, Joint Economic Committee, Congress of the United States, Washington 1969, p. 1205 (U.S. Government Printing Office).

From 1965 objectives were clarified and programmes were classified by objective, by target population group, and by the method of financing each programme element. The programmes were related to intermediary performance indicators, e.g. hospital area constructed. Analyses have been undertaken of the treatment for certain diseases, e.g. four types of cancer in order to establish, for a given expenditure, treatment for which type offers the greatest number of lives saved.

CONCLUSION

This paper has dealt with medical care from an economist's viewpoint. The author accepts that each doctor can be relied upon to provide the most appropriate treatment available for an individual patient. There is an economic problem however since the best that an individual doctor can do depends upon the resources, including his own time, available to him at a given time. The economic approach is one which seeks to ensure, for the whole population, that resources are being put to the best uses given the objectives. The various requirements for efficiency discussed are those to which the PPB system addresses itself. Whether or not developments in the economic management of medical care in Britain should lead to the PPB system found in the U.S.A. is an open question, but there can be little doubt that if the basic requirements for efficiency are met we shall have something which is, in fundamental respects, something like PPB.

COMMENT ON 'PROBLEMS OF EFFICIENCY'

A. J. CULYER
University of York

Mr Levitt's paper discusses a normative concept of efficiency which is restricted in two ways—one explicit and the other only implicit. The first is that he takes output objectives (somehow defined) as given in the context of the NHS. The second is that, following Arrow, his efficiency criterion is couched entirely in terms of 'ideals' rather than in terms of what degree of efficiency is possible under a broad spectrum of institutional services. In my comments I want to explore more fully the implications of both these restrictions with special emphasis on the central problem, namely that of getting information—a costly commodity without which we do not know what efficiency exists at any time or in any circumstances. It will be useful to treat each blade of the Marshallian scissors in turn.

DEMAND

Society's demand for health care may be conceptually divided into two parts. First, there is the sum of all individual demands for personal current treatment at current prices, and future availability of treatment at expected prices or current 'futures' prices. Second, there is the sum of all individual demands for current treatment and and future availability of treatment for *other people*. If we seek to know whether resources today are being assigned to uses for which they have the highest present values of utility, we need to know the sizes of all these four demands, which together comprise total benefit streams from health care provision, and which put a value dimension on *outputs* (cf. Levitt's list, p. 37).

Now consider how various alternative institutional devices might reveal some of these values. Consider first a community in which all social action is performed on the voluntary basis of individuals making binding contracts together whenever it was in their mutual interest. Individual demands for personal treatment, the evidence suggests, are most efficiently made in this way, either directly to suppliers or via insurance middlemen. As Arrow has shown, the abstract efficiency conventions require maximum discrimination according to risk, though in the presence of less than perfect information for patients and less than perfect competition among suppliers of services (enabling them, for instance, not to have to make maximum profits to its limited discriminations, or to pool risks, etc.) the achievement of the 'ideal' may be too costly (which means of course that the 'ideal' was not ideal). Institutions by which payment occurs at the time of receipt might be expected to cope with this reasonably well. (Well enough?)

Such institutions, however, would not cope so well with the current demand for future capacity. A person who, let us suppose, currently fails to insure himself, but later changes his mind, may find that the capacity in the future is not available. Since a future bed available for one is also a future bed for another, the individual finds himself in the familiar dilemma of the prisoner, which the institution just mentioned cannot deal with. An institution which could cope with this is voluntary prepayment, which would induce future capacity and would provide a mechanism by which the demands would be revealed. Well enough?

Neither of these two institutions could cope very well with the familiar type of externalities which arise in the personal consumption (or non-consumption) of health care. The means they offer for mutual contracts are too costly relative to the gains from such trading. In these cases it seems that the cheapest way of getting the preferences out into the open is via collective, rather than individual action. 'Politically' individuals might 'vote' to pay tax to subsidise (say) vaccination programmes, where the political unit appropriate would depend in part upon the geographical nature of the externality. Prisoners' dilemma problems remain however, so we may still ask how well this institution performs its task.

The second type of demand—that for care for other individuals—is not at all efficiently revealed by individual private contracting. Again, voluntary organisations of individuals for collective action appear to be the most effective method of providing (say) free care for the aged, the poor, for soldiers or for unmarried mothers, etc., though again the imperfections of such collective organisations whether they be private charitable groups or the largest conceivable political unit, are well-known, and largely the same difficulties apply to all these 'clubs'. Again practice falls short of the ideal. To think along these lines, however, indicates an appropriate role for public pressures in health resource allocation, and also suggests an *inappropriate* role. We thus have a preliminary way of tackling some of the questions posed by Mr Salter in his paper.

Levitt's dichotomy between the market and the state, while familiar, seems to me to be unproductive. If the objective is to detect increases in society's utility in the Paretian sense,[1] and if society is no more than the sum of all the individuals in it, the relevant question seems to me to be to seek that set of institutions which will do the job best, always remembering that institutions are none of them perfect and none of them free goods. Of Levitt's list of properties of an efficient system, 75% contain society's demand as an integral part, but in the latter part of the paper, this dimension is effectively buried and the 'state', which is presumably not the same as 'society' (or is it?) is assumed to know it all. However, it doesn't, as anyone who has had to try a bit of cost-benefit analysis for the 'state' knows only too well—as if it is not obvious anyway. One thing, however, has to be emphasised, and that is that it is simply not valid to observe that one institution is imperfect (as judged by some conceptual ideal of the perfect) and thence to conclude that another must necessarily be better. In an imperfect world we have to choose intelligently between imperfect (man-invented) institutions, and to do so we need all the information we can get about how they will work. One of the interesting things about the NHS type of system is that it generates practically no information at all about benefits, which at the operational stage makes the economist's job somewhat hard but fascinating since it tests his ingenuity in inventing surrogate measures of demand. But he should also test his ingenuity in inventing new institutions or variations on old ones to improve the revelation of relevant benefits.

[1] Meaning that if at least one person is better off as he sees it without anyone else being worse off, this is an increase in society's 'utility'. If some gain and others lose it does not mean that there is no improvement, only that we have no means of telling.

SUPPLY

Not surprisingly, therefore, Levitt's efficiency criterion is watered down to a 'least cost' one—and a rather special one at that—and he takes the outputs as settled. For the purposes of argument one may suppose that some mythical omniscient observer has decided them 'correctly'. The only costs which are admitted are fiscal expenditures net of contributions and charges. But since costs are the highest utility foregone by doing something, this seems to me to be a dubious procedure according to Mr Levitt's own methodological dicta. Furthermore, there is no questioning here of the possibility that fiscal cost and social cost may diverge, and yet we can all think of countless ways in which such divergences arise and ought to be allowed for. Levitt's single example in terms of relative factor intensities and a fixed supply of labour to the manufacturing sector, does not seem to me to be a convincing example of external costs—unless he is arguing that labour in the NHS is exploited.

Proposals for cost-effectiveness studies and for the estimation of health care production functions are sweet music to any economist's ears, and several of us are anxious to do more work in these areas, but fundamental problems still remain at the conceptual level which have to be settled in some way before principles get practised. Levitt has rightly observed that non-profit organisations in the market may signal false information about costs. But what validity ought to be placed on the cost information generated by non-profit organisations in the NHS? A cost function is supposed to be a least-cost function, but how reliable would econometrically estimated functions be as a guide to economic efficiency?

CONCLUSIONS

Levitt and I will almost certainly agree on one thing—we ought to make use of whatever information is available. We may not agree, however, on how much is desirable or what sorts are relevant. Taking the purpose of Levitt's paper at its face value—as a general methodological discussion of the meaning of efficiency and how it might be implemented—he has slid round too many corners for me to be happy. As a more restricted plea, however, for a continuation and increase in the application of quantitative techniques to increase efficiency in the public sector little bit by little bit, I thoroughly applaud him. Output budgeting (the use of cost-effectiveness techniques to choose between alternative means of achieving a given objective) has some fascinating possibilities within the context of the NHS. Output budgeting, however, does not take extant institutional arrangements for granted, as I have already tried to urge in a wider context that they should not be. Suppose, for example, that the PPB analyst wanted to study the prevention of disease in England and Wales. He would find that mass radiography was a Department of Health and Social Security responsibility, but expenditure on quarantine stations a responsibility of the Ministry of Agriculture, Fisheries and Food; that the Home Office makes a grant in aid to the National Society for the Prevention of Accidents, and that local authority expenditure on sewerage and sewage disposal comes out of Rate Support Grants of the central government. And so on. There is also lots of scope for economic ingenuity in inventing institutions of various kinds to get costs as well as benefits better revealed by individuals and establishments within the NHS. But we should not kid ourselves that by doing this kind of work we are necessarily improving efficiency in the sense that Levitt wants us to suppose that we are. The net needs to be cast far wider if that ambitious kind of claim is to be upheld. In short, I found the promise of the first page unfulfilled in what followed—which would not be so serious a fault if it were not a worrying inference I tend to draw that Levitt is elevating practical expediency to the status of methodological precept, rather than using the latter to make tomorrow's expediency better than today's.

EQUALITY IN THE NATIONAL HEALTH SERVICE:

INTENTIONS, PERFORMANCE AND PROBLEMS IN EVALUATION

M. H. COOPER
University of Exeter
and
A. J. CULYER
University of York

The National Health Service has been seen by many as the embodiment of the principle of access to health resources by those in need as a human right.[1] The mechanism by which this right was to be guaranteed was the nationalisation of health resources coupled with the removal of the price barrier from the acquisition of health care. With need established in principle as the sole criterion of allocation, only abuse remained as a problem. Thus, since 1948 committees of enquiry have, in the main, concerned themselves with the possibility of abuse rather than with the problem of defining or measuring adequacy. The assumption appears generally to have been that once these reforms became a reality more resources would be devoted to health care and that these resources would be inevitably more equitably distributed than would have been the case if health had been left in the private sector.

The assumption that public provision would necessarily lead to more resources in the health sector than might otherwise have been the case, has been frequently challenged in the past.[2] The evidence however, though consistent with the hypothesis that nationalisation reduces overall allocation to health care, is rather sketchy and circumstantial. Basically it lies in comparisons of relative percentages

[1] For persuasive statements of this view, see most of the works of R. M. Titmuss.
[2] An early and controversial example was D. S. Lees, *Health Through Choice*, Institute of Economic Affairs, London 1961.

of GNP devoted to health care between Britain and other countries of roughly comparable wealth, combined, where possible, with comparisons of relative provision and utilisation rates (e.g. consultation and hospitalisation rates). There are huge definitional problems inherent in such international comparisons although there is now growing evidence of variations for which an explanation is required. There are, for example, twice as many hospital-based surgeons *per capita* in the U.S.A. as in the U.K. Furthermore, these surgeons are performing twice as many operations. In addition, it is estimated that as many operations again are performed in the U.S.A. by doctors not holding surgical posts within hospitals. The uncomfortable, as distinct from the threatening, complaints figure more prominently in the U.S. statistics. Haemorrhoidectomy is performed three times more frequently on men, and five times more frequently on women in the U.S.A., and there are similar disparities in the rates for thyroidectomy, herniorrhaphy and hysterectomy. These contrasts seem the more surprising in a country known to have large medically deprived sections within its population. One possible explanation is, of course, that these disparities reflect not so much unmet need in the U.K. as the existence of 'unnecessary' operations in the U.S.A., although by no means all of the contrast is confined to the relatively trivial (e.g. operations performed on the eye).[3]

Much easier to refute is the more extravagant claim that the NHS has eliminated all medical need. At current prices the existence of excess demand for health care is prima facie evidence for a divergence from Paretian optimality, but if satisfying need replaces the Paretian criterion, such excess demands do not necessarily carry any normative connotation. Practical questions of what devices are used to allocate resources remain, however, as well as normative ones concerning which devices ought to be used and how much demand is to be met in any given period of time. The latter is equivalent to defining the operational meaning of need. The NHS clearly does not, and cannot, cater for need in the sense of providing resources sufficient to preserve all lives or to exploit fully all medical techniques. Scarcity of resources precludes such a conception of need.[4]

[3] See J. P. Bunker, *A Comparison of Operation and Surgical Manpower in the U.S. and in England and Wales*, Mimeo., Stanford University 1969.
[4] No doubt this misconception explains Aneurin Bevan's hope that the NHS would be a self-eliminating expense. Once the backlog of medical need had been met the health bill was predicted to be static for twenty years.

Even medical need, however, is itself a relative concept and cannot in practice be precisely determined in technical terms. With the decline in the importance of the acute infectious disorders, sickness is becoming increasingly a relative rather than an absolute concept. It is no longer typically the case that an individual is fit at 11 a.m., sick and in need of a doctor at 1 p.m., and possibly dead or on the way to recovery three days later. The stress disorders (e.g. respiratory disease and cancer) are chronic and their onset insidious. The moment of calling the doctor is a matter of personal judgement. The patient performs the first all-important diagnosis while, in marked contrast, the onset of most infectious diseases is all too obvious. Increasingly, new layers of sickness, as they are revealed or their treatment becomes a possibility, demand a new kind of health service and a new order of expense. They do not on the whole lend themselves to immediate medical success or failure, but rather to costly and repetitious medical servicing of faulty bodies. In short, equating marginal utilities with zero was, and still is, a practical impossibility.

The gap between what at any moment in time is technically feasible and what, in the context of competing claims upon resources, can be delivered to the patient apparently in need, is becoming increasingly obvious. This springs largely from the publicity recently afforded to such issues as whether or not to resuscitate elderly patients and to the unmet demands for heart, lung and kidney machines, for kidney and heart transplants and for a nationwide cervical cytology service. It is also the case that the British institutional framework has in reality produced lower utilisation rates (e.g. consultation and hospitalisation rates, etc.) than the American 'mixed' system. Clearly, rationing persists; the difference lies in the form that it takes. The danger is that, faced with a rising health bill, society searches for waste and abuse rather than attempts to assess whether the increase is simply a reflection of medical progress and/or consumers' demand or patients' need.

The debate concerning the relative virtues of the price mechanism as a method of allocation has tended to deflect interest away from the question of whether the removal of price has in fact resulted in a more equitable distribution of the available health resources (irrespective of their actual amount). The declared intent was that all the NHS or any part of it was to be available to everyone in England and Wales. The Act imposes no limitations based on financial means, age, sex, employment or vocation, areas of residence or insurance qualification.[5] 'It is intended that there shall be no limitation on the kind of medical assistance given.'[6] The remainder of this paper discusses the extent to which the actuality reflects just one of these intentions, namely that of geographical equality. It implies a clear and objective measure of variations in the extent to which need is met without requiring us to define individual need levels—definitions which have not been explicitly stated before in any case.

It is generally acknowledged that the stock of manpower and capital which the NHS inherited was very unequally distributed geographically (though detailed and systematic evidence is absent). Certainly the National Health Insurance Scheme, by omitting hospitalisation from its coverage, left the distribution of consultants virtually untouched between the two world wars. After World War II some counties lacked even a single gynaecologist, whilst in the eastern area only two hospitals could boast a psychiatrist and no thoracic surgeon or dermatologist was readily available at all.[7] Furthermore, although by 1938 the 'panel system' covered some 40% of the population, the distributing of purchasing power exerted a strong and predictable influence upon the location of general practitioners.

The inception of the NHS in 1948 did not bring in its wake any sweeping changes. The stock was taken over much as it stood and the evidence is that it remains very unequal to this day. The newly appointed regional hospital boards were instructed to assess the need for new resources and to secure 'a proper and sufficient service of all kinds for persons in their area'.[8] Aid by which to adjudge 'proper and sufficient' was provided by the Ministry in the form of ratios of specialists to population. These ratios proved so unrealistic that they were for all practical purposes stillborn.[9]

The introduction of geographically uniform rates of pay for hospital doctors and of uniform *per capita* payments for GPs left the

---

[5] *The National Health Service*, Cmnd. 6761, London 1946 (H.M.S.O.).

[6] *Hansard*, vol. 422, Col. 45, London, 30 April 1946 (A. Bevan).

[7] See The Nuffield Provincial Hospitals Trust, *The Hospital Surveys*, London 1946 (O.U.P.).

[8] *Ministry Circular*, R.H.B. 48, No. 1.

[9] Rosemary Stevens points out that according to these ratios there should have been 238 WTE consultants and SHMOs in physical medicine by 1962. In fact by 1966 there were still only 94. R. Stevens, *Medical Care in Modern England*, London 1966 (Yale University Press).

relative attractiveness of practising in pleasant areas of Britain and in centres of relative excellence largely intact. The right to treat private patients also remained as a further inducement to practise in these same areas.

In the case of GPs a process of negative direction was introduced. Some Executive Council areas were closed to new entrants, thus pushing them into under-doctored areas with over 2,500 patients to the average list. So long as the number of GPs was increasing this policy achieved a considerable degree of success. The population living in areas declared under-doctored fell from 52% in 1952 to 17% in 1961. But as the increase in doctors slowed down and then their numbers actually began to decline, this proportion increased again to 34%. Indeed the average list size is now slightly greater than it was in 1950.

Additions to the stock of hospital doctors have simply reflected the existing distribution. Only areas likely to attract new staff have advertised new posts, whilst there has been no positive attempt at direction from the centre or any inducements offered to attract talent to the less attractive areas.

Defining 'area of residence' at its broadest we have attempted to assess the extent of inequalities in both manpower and expenditure between the areas covered by each of the fifteen regional hospital boards. Thirty-one indices were constructed from official sources and are presented in the Appendix. It can be seen that in almost every instance the Sheffield Region appears less well endowed than the Oxford Region. Although it is frequently difficult meaningfully to interpret some of them they raise a great number of questions which are in urgent need of an answer. Why, for example, has the Newcastle Region twice as many gynaecologists per female as Sheffield; why has Birmingham twice as many whole-time equivalent consultants as Sheffield; why has Liverpool twice as many psychiatrists as Manchester? Six indices have ranges of over 100%, sixteen of over 50% and one a range of over 600%.

No evidence of one variable compensating for a deficiency in another could be found. The areas relatively deprived on one yardstick were not compensated on another. For example, the correlation coefficient between medical salaries per patient week and nursing salaries was 0·84; that between medical salaries and expenditure upon equipment, 0·73; and that between equipment and pharmaceuticals,

0·67. Nor was there any evidence of capital substitution for labour or vice versa.

To the extent that teaching hospitals with their superior staff/patient ratios and heavy concentrations of consultants with A+ distinction rewards are centres of excellence, it could be maintained on the equality of need criterion that access to their beds should also be equal irrespective of region. Indeed, Wessex has no such hospital beds while the North Western Metropolitan Region has one bed per 615 people. Excluding Wessex and all the Metropolitan area, the range is from Manchester with 3,714 persons per bed to Oxford with 1,356. There is, of course, undoubtedly a case to be made for centres of excellence as such, but for consistency, an egalitarian and well advertised set of allocation principles for patients drawn from a national catchment area is required. All should have equal opportunity of benefiting in accordance with medically determined need.

In the period since 1962, relative regional inequalities appear from a preliminary investigation to be increasing. The coefficient of variation for consultants per million population was 15% in 1962 and 17% in 1966 despite a 22% increase in their total numbers. Gynaecologists and obstetricians, for example, increased over the period by 11% but their coefficient of variation rose from 17% to 19%. Again the coefficient of variation for general practitioners rose from 18% to 21% but this time in the face of a fall in their numbers by 2·2%. Even in the case of consultants where manpower has been growing there does not appear to have been any systematic attempt to erase inequalities.

The NHS successfully dismantled the price barrier but has failed to deal with others. Inequalities of a geographical nature appear to be no more equitable than those resulting from inequalities in the distribution of purchasing power. There was nothing inherent in the 1946 Act which would have systematically brought equality about. Indeed even today the data upon which to base relevant decisions remain largely lacking. Richard Crossman recently described the problem of regional inequalities as the most difficult he had to face. The 'disparity was so big' that there was no easy way of aiding 'underprivileged areas with a major legitimate grievance' without cutting back on the more favoured areas.[10] Clearly good intentions,

[10] Reported in *The Guardian*, 27 November 1969.

even when they reflect the will of a majority of the electorate, are not enough.

This paper clearly implies more questions than it has attempted to answer. In particular, there are several fundamental problems relating to the application of economic techniques of analysis. One such problem evidently concerns the concept of need. Cost-effectiveness studies are one method which can be employed independently of value-judgements about the appropriateness of various rates of output of health services, and they have been and are being used at official levels. There may also, however, be a case for extending this kind of analysis to evaluate different objectives, or at least to rank them in terms of priorities, in a kind of systems analysis which might question the desirability or feasibility of egalitarianism. The adoption of any kind of allocation criterion based upon need also raises fundamental questions concerning the meaning of social cost. The methodology of cost-effectiveness analysis appears deceptively simple at the conceptual level (as distinct from practical difficulties) for if consumers' marginal valuations are rejected as a basis of allocating health resources on the demand side, their relevance may also be examined on the supply side as the basis for calculating social opportunity cost. The problem is even more intense if, for example, lost consumers' surpluses are included as costs of egalitarianism, for this reinstates marginal valuations of the health care services themselves as relevant in the choice of degree of equality, even if it does not imply their use as ultimate demand or need criteria.

A thorough-going rejection of consumers' valuations must imply their rejection on the supply side as well as for demand. But in this case one is apparently confronted with an absence of relevant economic techniques for deciding what constitutes efficiency even of the restricted sort. An asymmetrical rejection, however, raises important conceptual and methodological problems as to the meaning of costs. One way out of these difficulties would be to consider inequalities in health care consumption as externalities, which, while enabling economists to work with traditional tools of analysis, would also, however, question most commonly accepted concepts of need and would also throw open again the entire question of the appropriateness of nationalisation as an efficient means of their internalisation.

We have contented ourselves at this stage with looking at the extent of current inequalities. The questions of methodology need to be solved before it can be decided whether they ought to be eliminated, whether it is worth levelling up or down, or whether national rates of provision are currently too low or too high in either specific cases or regarding the health care complex as a whole. Less formal, but no less important, questions concern the means by which resources are currently allocated in practice in the face of excess demand and queues, and the extent to which techniques for discrimination between competing claimants can be invented which are consistent with objectives for equal territorial physical provision.

Appendix. Indices of Regional Variation

	Range for England & Wales, excluding Metropolitan Regions			Range for England & Wales, including Metropolitan Regions			Coefficient of Variation excluding Metropolitan Regions	Two regional examples	
	1 Most Favourable	2 Most unfavourable	3 Larger as % of Smaller	4 Most Favourable	5 Most unfavourable	6 Larger as % of Smaller	7 %	8 Oxford	9 Sheffield
MANPOWER									
1. Population per WTE consultant	4,425	8,932	202	4,425	8,932	202	16·81	6,315	8,932
2. Population per hospital doctor-medical assistant or below	3,355	6,140	183	2,283	6,140	269	16·86	3,761	6,140
3. Population per GP (principals only)	1,593	3,685	231	n.a.	n.a.	n.a.	20·93	2,352	2,825
PHYSICAL FACILITIES									
4. Staffed beds allocated per 1,000 population	10·81	7·64	141	13·77	7·64	182	10·86	8·32	7·64
5. Mean daily beds available per 1,000 population	10·73	7·54	143	13·59	7·54	182	10·87	8·17	7·54
UTILISATION									
6. Mean daily bed occupation per 1,000 population	9·15	6·73	136	6·73	11·69	174	10·99	6·73	6·41
7. Cases treated (deaths & discharges) per 1,000 population	120·0	85·3	141	120·7	85·3	141	9·95	109·7	85·3
8. Utilisation of bed capacity (6 divided by 4)	84·8	80·9	105	80·9	84·9	105	1·53	80·9	83·8
9. Mean waiting time (weeks)	13·0	16·6	128	13·0	16·6	128	8·05	15·4	16·6
10. Median waiting time (weeks)	8·6	12·1	141	8·5	12·1	142	10·68	11·4	12·1
11. Persons waiting per 1,000 population	8·1	14·6	180	8·1	14·6	180	18·46	12·7	11·3
12. Mean length of stay per spell of illness in days	14·4	18·6	129	14·4	19·3	134	7·31	14·4	16·7

Appendix. Indices of Regional Variation

	Range for England & Wales, excluding Metropolitan Regions			Range for England & Wales, including Metropolitan Regions			Coefficient of Variation excluding Metropolitan Regions	Two regional examples	
	1 Most Favourable	2 Most unfavourable	3 Larger as % of Smaller	4 Most Favourable	5 Most unfavourable	6 Larger as % of Smaller	7 %	8 Oxford	9 Sheffield
EXPENDITURE									
13. Expenditure per in-patient week of medical salaries and wages as a % of the national mean	135·2	88·4	154	135·2	88·4	154	12·32	135·2	105·1
14. Expenditure per in-patient week of nursing salaries and wages as a % of the national mean	112	90	125	112	90	125	6·07	112	102
15. Expenditure per in-patient week on pharmaceuticals as a % of the national mean	108	84·0	128	108	84	128	6·81	108	98·5
16. Expenditure per in-patient week on medical and surgical equipment as a % of the national mean	137		189	137	72	189	15·84	137	109
17. Expenditure per in-patient week on catering as a % of the national mean	107·5	82·0	132	113·1	82·0	137	7·48	107·5	105·7
18. Expenditure on psychiatric hospitals *per capita* per annum (mental illness and mental subnormality), £	3·1	1·8	172	4·7	1·7	278	34·11	2·2	1·9
19. Expenditure in hospitals *per capita* per annum, £	10-20	7·22	141	10-20	7·22	141	11·48	7·76	7·20
QUALITATIVE INDICES									
20. % hospital medical staff at medical assistant or below, born overseas	32	54	169	29·8	54	186	17·76	38	54
21. % hospital medical staff at medical assistant or below in non-teaching hospitals, born overseas	35	66	189	35	66	189	19·15	49	66
22. A+ award holders as % WTE consultants	2·2	0·3	714	n.a.	n.a.	n.a.	71·82	2·2	0·3

Appendix. Indices of Regional Variation

	Range for England & Wales, excluding Metropolitan Regions			Range for England & Wales, including Metropolitan Regions			Coefficient of Variation excluding Metropolitan Regions	Two regional examples	
	1 Most Favourable	2 Most unfavourable	3 Larger as % of Smaller	4 Most Favourable	5 Most unfavourable	6 Larger as % of Smaller	7 %	8 Oxford	9 Sheffield
23. A award holders as % WTE consultants	3·7	1·9	196	n.a.	n.a.	n.a.	20·26	2·2	2·8
24. B award holders as % WTE consultants	9·2	7·3	127	n.a.	n.a.	n.a.	8·41	8·8	7·3
25. C award holders as % WTE consultants	19·0	14·7	130	n.a.	n.a.	n.a.	9·25	18·2	15·9
26. % of GP principals with lists less than 1,600	15·0	7·2	208	n.a.	n.a.	n.a.	29·67	7·2	8·0
27. % of GP principals with lists over 3,000	9·7	29·8	307	n.a.	n.a.	n.a.	40·37	19·4	29·8
WTE CONSULTANTS BY SELECTED SPECIALITY									
28. Anaesthetists per million population	22·9	13·6	169	23·6	13·6	172	14·96	18·4	13·6
29. Gynaecologists and obstetricians per million female population	21·7	11·0	197	22·6	11·0	205	18·83	15·0	11·0
30. Consultants treating mental illness per million population	16·3	8·5	192	23·2	8·5	270	16·46	14·6	11·8
31. Consultants treating subnormality per million population	4·2	1·1	385	4·2	1·1	385	41·61	2·6	2·2

Sources:

1, 2: Ministry of Health, Tables R1 and R2, London 1966.
3: Ministry of Health, London.
4, 5, 6, 7, 11: *Hospital Returns* (Form S.H.3) 1967, and the Ministry of Health, London.
8: *Hospital Returns* (Form S.H.3) 1967.
9, 10, 12: Ministry of Health and General Registrar Office, *Report on Hospital In-Patient Enquiry for the Year 1967*, London 1968, Table 6A (H.M.S.O.).
13, 14, 15, 16, 17: Ministry of Health, *Hospital Costing Returns*, Year Ended March 31, 1965, London 1965 (H.M.S.O.).
18, 19: Ministry of Health, *Hospital Costing Returns*, Year Ended March 31, 1967, London 1967 (H.M.S.O.).
20, 21: Ministry of Health, Table R2, London 1966.
22, 23, 24, 25: Ministry of Health, *Annual Report 1966*, London 1967 (H.M.S.O.).
26, 27: *Ibid.*, Table 8.
28, 29, 30, 31: As for 1 and 2.

COMMENT ON 'EQUALITY IN THE NATIONAL HEALTH SERVICE:

INTENTIONS, PERFORMANCE AND PROBLEMS IN EVALUATION'

G. R. FORD

Department of Health and Social Security

If equality or inequality within the NHS are to be demonstrated and commented upon, it seems essential to look first of all at the indices that are used. The Appendix shows that these have been divided into groups: manpower, physical facilities, utilisation, expenditure, 'qualitative' indices and WTE consultants by selected specialty. One of these groups purports to give indices of quality but the only one which seems to me to be valuable is the percentage of GP principals with lists over 3,000. Apart from line 13 the indices of expenditure do not demonstrate very great differences between Oxford and Sheffield and nor do they cast Sheffield in an unfavourable light compared with the national mean. The figures for utilisation again only show a marked difference in the cases treated (deaths and discharges) per 1,000 of the population (and crude population is probably an inexact measure of needs). Demand as defined by Spek (demand = that part of the need for care which is represented by those individuals who come into the system for consultation and treatment and who are willing to wait) is not manifestly different. However although lines 9, 10 and 11 do not show a great difference of unmet demand in Sheffield compared with Oxford, it is accepted that figures for waiting times are related to supply and there may be unmet need.

Nevertheless the first two indices—the population per WTE consultant and the population per hospital doctor—are clear indications of inequality in the distribution of specialist services, which is surprising in a system which has been in action for twenty years and where there has been a real effort, particularly in the last ten years, to even up medical manpower differences. The authors state that in the period since 1962 regional inequalities have been increasing. This is alarming. Since 1962 the Advisory Committee on Consultant Establishments has paid particular attention to regional differences in consultant staffing in every speciality. Norms have been established with the object of raising the staffing level in comparatively under-manned areas. Moreover the Department of Health and Social Security controls senior registrars and registrar establishments. In spite of central control of new medical posts the situation is said to have got worse rather than better. What more can be done? Is the defect in the allocation of resources, both medical manpower and funds, related to the small amount of unbespoke resources which is all that the Department has at its disposal? In the case of manpower this is new posts, and in the case of funds it is the new money avail-able each year, which is only a small proportion of the 'fixed' revenue allocation. The strongest influence on allocation of money between regions is apparently the existing fabric, i.e. capital developments and associated personnel. It is possible that the inequality between regions has been exacerbated because the rationing process (or perhaps one should say the rationalisation process) has not been imposed strictly enough, a procedure which might necessarily involve closure of facilities and direction of labour. Rationing itself has occasionally brought unlooked-for benefits in its train. Applied to food during the war it brought about a higher standard of nutrition when rationing ended the standard of nutrition dropped, taking five or six years to recover once again to wartime levels. An example nearer home is the short supply of hospital beds which gave rise to early ambulation after surgery, preparatory to discharge home. This had undoubted therapeutic advantages as distinct from hospital utilisation advantages. No doubt there are also disadvantages which are equally significant.

It is possible to look at the apparent inequalities in a different way and to measure what is being done, cheaply, in one region and com-pare this with what is being done expensively in another? It may be that there is a basic bread-and-butter service in some areas while others go in for jam.

Perhaps more important is the need to devise measures for alloca-tion of funds based on good demographic data, and knowledge of the factors that influence utilisation/need of health resources. We know that the age/sex structure of the population is one important factor, but others—social class, educational attainments, income—together with environmental factors such as the level of industrialisation, are probably important too.

Is it possible that planners of the future may use more refined indices of the need for health services?

In Sweden such factors are being measured. Not only do they know that 20% of the population use 80% of the health resources but they appear to be very near to being able to know who this particularly disadvantaged group are. It is at least possible that different ways of meeting those needs could be devised.

The authors of the paper discuss the fact that the usual reaction to increased costs of health services is a search for abuse of the existing system rather than an acceptance that increased costs may indeed represent increased need. In my opinion there has indeed been concern about *under*-use of the health service. Examples are (i) the suspected restraint by elderly age groups in their use of available services; (ii) the lack of use of the cervical cytology service by those most at risk. In the United States, as the authors point out, tissue committees were set up to prevent *abuse*. While up to now this aspect of wrong use of services does not appear to have received much attention, certainly at local level, peer review of the type already discussed by Dr Draper may carry out this function. Rising costs obviously have to be reviewed in terms of increased need and of resource allocation—possibly with a view to reallocation.

Concluding that geographical inequality exists and cannot easily be remedied by the levelling measures at the Department's disposal, including capital investment, indices of unmet need or morbidity and mortality figures seem to be necessary to validate the conclusions that this inequality is associated with poor results from medical care. At the same time more rational planning both of ways of providing the service (community and hospital-located services) and of the actual distribution of services in relation to factors of age, industry, social class, etc., seems desirable and could surely be hastened by economic analysis of the problems involved.

A MODEL OF THE MEDICAL CARE SYSTEM:

A GENERAL SYSTEMS APPROACH

D. L. CROMBIE

Director, Research Unit,
Royal College of General Practitioners

PART I. THE MODEL

Any rational debate about deployment of resources within the health services should logically begin with consideration of models of the system.

The main aim of any system of medical care is to help the patient, as an individual or community of individuals, to solve or ameliorate their clinical problems. These problems have physical, emotional and socio-economic components (Crombie, 1963b). Their solution may or may not involve the formal diagnosis of some disease process (Crombie, 1963c, d) and the patient may not even be aware that he has a problem.

Medical care has three main dimensions (Fig. 1):

1. The most fundamental of all is the clinical split into assessment processes and therapeutic processes; the other two dimensions are secondary to this.
2. The second is the operational split into domiciliary and hospital-based services.
3. The third is the organisational split into individual and community requirements.

The assessment process which includes prognosis is split into symptomatic and presymptomatic levels and the therapeutic process is split into preventive and curative measures.

Medical Economics
The aim of all medical care must be to bring the maximum benefit

61

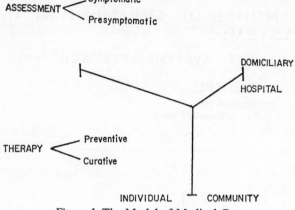

Figure 1. The Model of Medical Care

to the patient within limitations set by restricted resources. This is the only absolute value or principle in medical care. All other so-called 'principles' are *ad hoc* generalisations appropriate to some more limited problem situation, whether clinical, social, economic, organizational or ethical, and then only for the time being. In deploying the limited resources, the priorities must be determined by the relative effort expended (i) on the assessment of the problem, as compared with the action taken to deal with it, (ii) in 'prevention' as compared with 'cure', (iii) in the treatment of symptomatic illness as compared with presymptomatic illness, (iv) in the potential benefits to one patient compared with all other patients, and finally (v) in the deployment of resources from a centralised hospital base compared with the more diffused domiciliary services.

The quality of human existence in general depends primarily on the quality with which life problems are first assessed and then dealt with. Similarly, the quality of medical care depends primarily on the quality with which the patient's problems are first assessed and then dealt with. Assessment means more than establishing a formal diagnosis. Dealing appropriately with the problem means more than formal therapy.

The Assessment Process
In any rational system of medical care, assessment must precede therapy. Our system of medical care only works as effectively as it

does because of the presence of GPs who act as the primary assessors of previously undifferentiated clinical situations. They are greatly aided in the fulfilment of this situation by the secondary role of personal doctor which enables them to bring much data to the assessment and decision-making process which would not be accessible in any other way.

As the Horders' diagram illustrates (Fig. 2), the medical services deal with only a small proportion (25%) of the aberrations of health which people recognise in themselves (Horder and Horder, 1954).

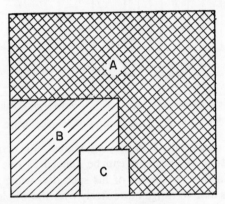

Figure 2. Total Morbidity and Medical Services
A. Total morbidity (100%).
B. Morbidity brought to general practitioners (25%).
C. Morbidity dealt with at hospital (3%–5%).

Again, of those who consult a medical practitioner, only a very small proportion (10–20%) are referred to hospital or specialist care. (A very small proportion indeed go direct to hospital.) These facts should induce a sense of humility in all who practise medicine.

The medical requirements of those who come to a practitioner (group B in Figure 2) are provided as shown in Figure 3. The left-hand square shows the allocation of total medical knowledge and techniques to the various specialties and to general practice. General practice requires a wide knowledge of techniques from all specialties, plus knowledge unique to general practice itself. This includes background information about the patient's past medical history, his social and financial situation, his personality, and the way he deals with the problems of life in general and disease in particular. The

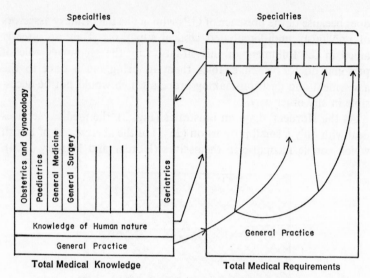

Figure 3. The Distribution of Medical Care

GP shares, with specialists, in varying degrees, a general knowledge of human nature. A specialist can be defined as one whose work remains within the boundaries of his specialty, while a consultant, like the GP, is able to range more freely over the whole of medicine (Crombie, 1963a).

The reason for this apportionment of knowledge becomes apparent when we consider the patients' needs and the ways in which they may be satisfied.

The right-hand square is approximately the same as area B in Figure 2. The important point here is that the GP, with only some 10% (or less) of total medical knowledge, is able to deal effectively with 80–90% of all medical problems. At the same time he is able to redirect, equally effectively, the remaining 10–20% of patients who require specialist services. He is able to combine these functions by virtue of his unique personal knowledge of each individual, in a relatively stable cohort of individuals with whom he remains in contact over many years. In my own practice, where, on average, 8% of the patients leave and a further 8% join each year, nearly 70% have been patients for ten years or more.

The doctor's personal knowledge certainly assists him in his function of assessor of needs, and any other practitioner who attempts to assess needs becomes, for the time being, a 'general practitioner'. Thus, a specialist in paediatrics or internal medicine to whom the public has direct access must become his own GP.

The present system in effect places the whole load of initial assessment on GPs, and most of the therapeutic load as well. To be preferred, any other system must be shown to be an improvement on this. The *essential* function is assessment; but the fact that simplification more often occurs in therapy than in assessment has enabled the GP to maintain his position as the main therapist in most branches of medicine, including psychiatry, paediatrics, geriatrics and dermatology. For obvious reasons he has almost wholly relinquished therapeutic activity in surgery, while retaining less and less in obstetrics.

PART II. THE PRIMARY ASSESSMENT AND RE-ASSESSMENT PROCESS IN CLINICAL MEDICINE

ASSESSMENT IN GENERAL PRACTICE

The first thing a GP has to decide is the relative importance of the emotional and physical factors in his patients' problems. Only the GP approaches the matter quite in this way, and his ability to do so depends on his unique previous knowledge of the patient. Where this knowledge is denied to the doctor, assessment has to be made by the more devious and less certain method of evaluating the emotional component by exclusion of the organic. This method of estimating the emotional component is clumsy. For the 10–20% of selected problems which reach the hospital-based doctor, it is suitable; but in general practice it is unsuitable and also wasteful of medical resources.

The organic element is less definable in illness encountered by GPs than it is in the selected illness encountered in hospital practice. The emotional element, on the other hand, is relatively more important in general practice. At hospital level, the clinical material includes serious organic disease with a relatively smaller recognised emotional content, and a satisfactory diagnosis in morphological and aetiological terms is therefore more likely.

The Total Clinical Assessment Load

The total clinical assessment load on general practice has been measured directly and indirectly in many ways.

C

The largest published source of data is the National Morbidity Survey carried out by the Registrar General's Office and the Royal College of General Practitioners in 1954 (Logan 1953, 1956; Logan and Cushion, 1958a, b). This was a study of all illness encountered in a representative population of Great Britain, numbering 250,000 people, over the course of one year. These were the patients of 170 recording doctors. The General Register Office, the College of General Practitioners and the Department of Health and Social Security are now co-operating in a further National Morbidity Survey to be held in 1970–71. This study will produce data comparable with that collected in the first study but will include a large range of other data, particularly about therapeutic habits, as well as diagnosis.

The bias recording systems which have been evolved in the Research Unit of the Royal College of General Practitioners are all directed toward their application to the measurement of the total clinical assessment load occurring in the recording practices. The recording methods and the data which is recorded are standardised. These recording systems, and their other applications, are described in detail later.

The Differentiation of the Physical, Emotional and Socio-Economic Components of Illness

The actual contribution of the social and welfare services within the total health care system has been measured in a study carried out by the Research Unit of the Royal College of General Practitioners in Stoke. The individual services rendered by these welfare and social services to those provided by the rest of the health service are in the ratio of 1:12·5.

The actual emotional content of the clinical problems brought to medical care has always been difficult to estimate, largely because we bring a uni-dimensional classification of disease to the labelling of the patient's condition. This Procrustean bed leads to estimates for the percentage of patients consulting with illnesses which are primarily emotional; they vary from 5 to 36% (Ryle, 1960).

Practitioners were asked to use a two-dimensional, five-point scale (Table 1) in which to allocate patients (Crombie, 1963b).

This enables an assessment to be made which is realistic. Although the subjective element must vary from practitioner to practitioner,

Table 1. Assessment of Emotional and Organic Elements in Disease

	I	II	III	IV	V
% of Episodes	52	21	13	6	8

   i. An illness all, or nearly all, organic
   ii. An illness mainly organic, but with some ab-
       normal emotional content
   iii. An illness with emotional and organic compon-
       ents in equal proportion
   iv. An illness mainly emotional, but with some
       organic content
   v. An illness all, or nearly all, emotional

the results are reasonably consistent. On average, the emotional element was at least as important as the organic in 27% of all illnesses encountered by these practitioners, and was appreciable in a further 21%. The discrepancy between these figures and the usually accepted figure of 5–10% is a measure of the distortion introduced by current medical nomenclature.

This point is laboured simply to show how indissoluble is any assessment process of physical and emotional components of illness, if it is going to be satisfactory. It is no use prosecuting vigorously the treatment of a patient's real but irrelevant backache when his clinical problem is severe depression. In our culture, it is still conventional to bring an organic 'handle' to the medical care system whenever the patient feels ill or diseased.

Generalist or Specialist Assessors

The case for the primary assessment of previously undifferentiated clinical material to be carried out by one person for each patient as presented in the previous section, has been based on two main arguments. The first is the need to assess at an early stage the emotional and organic components of any clinical problem. The second is the need for this assessment to be based not only on the integrated cerebral mechanisms of one assessing brain, but also on a network of essential prior personal information about the patient to which that brain must have access. The arguments in support of this second point must be more subjective than for the first, but some insight can be gained from the results of a recent study by the Research Unit and the Practice Organisation Committee of the Royal College of General Practitioners: *The Source of Information used in Clinical Decision-making.*

The results of this preliminary study make it clear that general practitioners in Great Britain, at least in their clinical decision-making, rely mainly on information generated *de novo* during the process of clinical problem-solving, either at the first consultation or as a result of that first consultation. It also makes it clear that most of the information already included in conventional record systems is largely redundant.

The clinical dialogue between the practitioner and the patient, on which the assessment is based, is equivalent to the logic branching systems on which computer-assisted diagnostic programmes are based. However, the personal doctor brings a personalised logic branching programme to each diagnostic situation. I would suggest, but cannot yet objectively substantiate, that the personal recorded notes of the practitioner are a set of nodes from which clinical assessment, highly appropriate to the specific patient, can spring for the problems which the patient may meet in the future.

Examples of these nodes are comments such as 'fussy wife', 'dirty house', 'drinks too much', 'always complains of physical illness when depressed', and so on. These highly selected and appropriate nodes, interacting with other information in the practitioner's mind, will provide the basis for generating an enormous range of *ad hoc* background information about any patient who has been a patient for any length of time.

Comparative Studies of the Relative Efficiency and Cost of Primary Assessment by Individuals with Differing Training and Skills

There is another argument, not confined to this section, in favour of a unitary assessor. This concerns the valuation of the individual as an individual *vis-à-vis* his group system or subsystems of his group system. It would seem, on the face of it, increasingly difficult to provide the necessary bias in this assessment valuation toward the individual by a system in which the assessment process is shared between a multiplicity of assessors. The only effective system based on a multiplicity of assessors is one where the whole problem area is fully structured, where the demarcation between different problem areas is clear-cut and where there is not only the minimum of overlap between assessment areas but even more important, no large gaps between the areas. This initial section has been elaborated in some detail to establish the point that this demarcation does not yet exist in medicine for the primary assessment of previously undifferentiated clinical material.

However, McKeown (1963) has suggested that some of these problems could be resolved by allocating the primary assessment to a set of specialist primary assessors. He has suggested that community care devolves not on generalist primary assessors, as at present, but on terms consisting of: paediatricians who look after all children up to 14; geriatricians who look after all those over 65; obstetricians who look after all women, not only during their pregnancies but also when they have any gynaecological disorder; and finally, general physicians who will deal with all the other problems of patients in the age group 15–64. The rationale of these proposals derives from the supposition that specialisation in a limited problem field would improve the quality of care provided by any individual doctor.

There are many arguments for and against the two alternatives of primary generalists *vis-à-vis* specialists which will not be considered in detail here. However, the contribution which the different systems might make to a lightening of the hospital load and the relative gain in therapeutic efficiency which may result from specialisation, compared with any loss in the quality of overall prior assessment of the clinical problems, are all of obvious importance. The Royal College of General Practitioners is planning studies to evaluate these two systems.

The Non-Medical Primary Assessor

The case for primary assessment to be based on one person has so far been based, in its turn, on the assumption that the assessor must be medically qualified. Could primary assessment be carried out as effectively by non-medically-qualified personnel?

Systems of primary assessment based on nurses are in operation now in Scandinavia. They are also used in this country in industry during working hours as primary assessors to the workers in many large industrial concerns. A study (unpublished) in a large electrical concern in Edinburgh in 1968, carried out by the Research Unit and the Practice Organisation Committee of the Royal College of General Practitioners, showed that in 1,000 representative episodes of illness during working hours dealt with by two nurses as primary assessors, 95% were assessed and therapy initiated without reference to the work's medical officer. In 3·5% of those referred to the medical officer the assessment and therapy suggested by the nurse were simply approved, and in only 2·5% of the total was any further direct action by the medical officer necessary. These figures are in contrast to previous estimates by doctors and nurses themselves of the work of the GP which nurses *believed* they could competently carry out as primary assessors. These figures (Crombie and Cross, 1957; Working Party, Royal College of General Practitioners, 1969; Hodgkin and Gillie, 1968) all give estimates nearer to 20% than 95%. This is, in any case, a misleading figure. In the study by Crombie and Cross (1957), for the 16% of the episodes in which it was assessed that a nurse could have been fully responsible for assessment and treatment, were the least serious and accounted for only 4% of the GP's total working time.

In the same study it was assessed that the nurse could have assisted with a further 24% of episodes with an additional, theoretical maximal saving of a further 15% of time. However, much of this saving would have been lost in the delegation process and it seems, from subsequent studies, that a doctor may, on many occasions, work much more quickly than a nurse (Hodgkin and Gillie, 1968).

There is no doubt that the discrepancy between these figures of 95–97·5% on the one hand and 4–28% on the other, reflect the inbuilt attitudes and values of doctors and nurses. The lower figure is what nurses who have never been put in the position of primary assessors *think* they could do. The higher figure reflects what a nurse actually *does* when given the job and full responsibility. The higher figure is, however, an underestimate to the extent that an unknown number of workers kept their problems for their own GPs when they thought that they were beyond the capacity of the nurse. We believe this figure to be relatively small but, until we have completed a further more detailed study to take this into account, we cannot be sure. We are also not sure whether the nurse's assessment was as adequate as assessment by a medically-qualified doctor might have been. Further studies in this field are proceeding and in plan.

Symptomatic and Presymptomatic Diagnosis
The appropriateness of presymptomatic over symptomatic diagnosis only arises for those conditions which fulfil the following criteria:

there is some therapeutic advantage from early diagnosis; there is some screening procedure which will identify all, or a large majority of, those individuals and only those individuals needing this preventive treatment in the presymptomatic phase; there is no overwhelming economic bar to implementing this screening; and the screening procedure can be accommodated within the spectrum of good clinical care without distorting it. Wilson and Jungfer (1967), in the most comprehensive review to date, define the procedure as 'the presumptive identification of unrecognised disease or defect by the application of tests, examinations or other procedures which can be applied rapidly. Screening tests sort out apparently well persons who probably have a disease from those who probably do not. A screening test is not intended to be diagnostic. Persons with positive or suspicious findings must be referred to their physicians for diagnosis and necessary treatment.'

At a recent symposium on presymptomatic diagnosis (Symposium on Presymptomatic Diagnosis, 1966) some of these problems were discussed. Without going into detail it is fair to say that no screening procedure fulfils all these criteria without qualifications. For example, cervical smear campaigns may be detecting the more slow-growing, less lethal carcinomata and tending to miss the virulent, rapidly growing and metastasising tumours. Tonometry in the screening for glaucoma produces a large proportion of false positives and fails to discover a significant proportion of those with the disease.

For some years it has been evident that mass detection drives for discovering diabetes based on discovery of glycosuria are appropriate only for highly selected at-risk groups (Royal College of General Practitioners, 1962, 1963). It has been pointed out (Crombie, 1964) that routine detection should be confined to those over 50 in the high-risk groups: i.e. individuals who are or have been obese, women who have borne more than six children or a baby weighing 10 lb or more at birth and those who have close relatives who are known diabetics. It was also pointed out that, far more important than this restricted screening, was the necessity for the GP to be aware of the possibility of diabetes during his routine contacts with his patients. In this particular example, where the conclusions were based on the mass detection drive carried out by the College Working Party, the numerical evaluation of the results lead us back, not to mass detection drives as such but to current good clinical practice. This consists in testing for glycosuria in all patients with certain disabilities such as vague ill health, peripheral vascular disease, or neuropathy particularly associated with ulceration of sepsis of the lower limbs, visual defects, coronary artery or cerebrovascular disease, vulvitis and balanitis.

The lack of knowledge about the natural history of many other diseases, including hypertension and ischaemic heart disease as the commonest and most important, also precludes them as candidates for any mass screening at present. In the example of ischaemic heart diseases, predisposition can be estimated (Morris, Kegan and Pattison, 1966), but is not suitable as a means for mass screening.

The lesson from all these examples is that we should be spending such limited resources as we have, not on half-baked screening campaigns but on intensive epidemiological studies of the natural history of these conditions, coupled with therapeutic trials where these are indicated.

Procedures which fulfil the criteria, such as screening for phenylketonuria and for congenital dislocation of the hip, exemplify other problems. In the first, the screening can be carried out by non-medically-qualified personnel, but abnormality is unlikely to exceed one in 10,000 births. The second example is of a commoner disease. However, the requisite examinations can easily become part of normal diagnostic ritual, applied at one of the many opportunities provided by routine contact with babies during the first twelve months of life. Testing for rhesus antibodies routinely during antenatal care is a second similar example, though antenatal care as a whole provides other lessons. It exemplifies the relative rapidity with which an appropriate diagnostic and preventive ritual can be formulated when it derives from an academic basis.

The ultimate fulfilment of this ritualisation process in the paediatric field can be epitomised by the paediatric record card devised by Dr J. N. Wright in collaboration with the Research Unit of the Royal College of General Practitioners. Not only is this card an example of a rational clinical balance between information needed for symptomatic and presymptomatic diagnosis, but for preventive medicine vis-à-vis curative medicine. It is also an example of a structured record to which all members of a primary assessment team in the community could contribute, with general indications as to who should contribute and when, as well as what they should contribute.

This card is, in effect, a basis for a medical care system from birth to the end of the fourth year of life, and the principle could be extended throughout life. This extension has not yet been attempted simply because the necessary information on which to make decisions about what is worth putting in is not yet available. These problems are dealt with in later sections.

We can summarise by saying that presymptomatic diagnosis has limited clinical application at present and requires an intensive research effort to establish its true place in clinical practice.

Not only must the effectiveness of screening programmes be proved, but ways of integrating these programmes into the present assessment systems of general practice must be devised. This integration must not distort these systems which are the most complex and efficient preventive and screening programmes in existence.

It is obvious that this is a field requiring intensive study, if we are to get an objective basis for rational decision-making, and I do not apologise for spending so much time in this area.

PREVENTIVE AND CURATIVE MEDICINE
The other main functional dimension of the medical care system, complementary to clinical assessment, concerns therapeutic action. Much less need be said about this in the context of the present debate.

The Total Therapeutic Load
The arguments for a single primary assessor developed in the first section do not apply to therapeutic action. The whole concept of successful medical specialism makes this clear. However, it was pointed out that much therapeutic activity is unsophisticated in its technical content and can be encompassed by the primary general assessor. A degree of therapeutic specialisation, say, in psychiatry, obstetrics, dermatology, paediatrics, in the long-term care of chronic disabling conditions at any age, in diabetes, in rheumatic conditions and, possibly, in ophthalmology, are all possible within a group practice based on otherwise conventional lines. *Conventional*, in this context, applies to the basis of generalist primary assessors. However, this specialisation would always be partial, both in the depth to which specialism in any one field can be taken by a general practitioner and to the range of specialisation that could be covered by

the twelve or twenty partners in any one group practice. This type of *ad hoc*, localised specialisation would never obviate the need for more conventional specialists in the same field, particularly where care involved the use of hospital beds.

The Place of the Therapeutic Generalists vis-à-vis a Specialist

The Place of Non-Medical Ancillaries in Therapy
This restriction will also apply to the system of general practice specialisation proposed by McKeown and already described. This system, when compared with conventional general practice, must be judged primarily on the relative efficiency of the primary assessment process and, secondarily, on the efficacy of therapeutic action in the two settings.

Any contribution to the hospital load by either system will be marginal. Such a comparison will be part of a larger comparative study to be carried out in Birmingham by the Study Practice of the Research Unit of the Royal College of General Practitioners. Included in this comparison will be an assessment of the different ways of delivering obstetric care, of utilising ancillary help of all kinds, of using hospital facilities (including staff, beds and other services) and of the integration of hospital and community services as a whole in the two settings.

The Relative Effectiveness and Cost of Preventive and Prophylactic Procedures vis-à-vis Traditional Curative Medicine
Studies in this field include an assessment of various potentially preventive procedures. However, as with presymptomatic diagnosis, prevention seems to be already included either in conventional clinical practice or in conventional immunisation and public health campaigns. For example, the preventive aspect is evident in the way in which GPs use antibiotics in the treatment of respiratory and urinary infections (Crombie, 1968).

The preventive element is also evident in other ways: in the way in which the GP uses oral diuretics to reduce, if not prevent attacks of acute left-sided heart failure, in his advice to the obese, the heavy smoker and drinker, and the patient with a family history of diabetes; in genetic counselling; in the handling of patients with emotional problems, inadequate personalities or with a history of previous psychiatric problems; and in his advice to women who wish to use oral contraceptives. The range of these preventive measures and the opportunities for initiating them stem from the continuity of the relationship between the GP and the majority of his patients, and from the fact that the patient traditionally initiates the consultation. Only GPs are aware of the volume and importance of the preventive work which they do. Its effects cannot at present be easily measured numerically; it is integrated into a pattern of medical care evolving gradually over the years and empirically absorbing diagnostic and therapeutic advances. In a workload study (Crombie and Cross, 1964) it was estimated that the percentages of time spent in contact with the patient at surgery and in the patient's home was as follows: assessing, 58%; advising, 23%; prescribing, 7%; therapeutic listening, 8%; and preventing, 4%. The opportunities which each GP has of clinical contact—on average five times with some 70% of his patients in each year—and the frequency and continuity of such contacts, including especially those which take place in the patient's home, enables the GP to identify at the earliest possible moment the emotionally disturbed patient who presents his problem as physical illness. There is an element of assessment in all therapy; and the good GP treats every contact with his patient as an opportunity to anticipate or forestall trouble.

This last section has ignored the more formal, conventional and systematic preventive or prophylactic element in general practice, which includes mass immunisation and inoculation campaigns and public health measures in general. These need not involve the GP, or other medically-qualified personnel in short supply, in much extra work, if he has adequate ancillary help. This applies to a lesser extent to antenatal care, possibly the most important systematised preventive component in GP care, and also to well-baby clinics.

Though the approach as outlined here is in its entirety an ideal, it is achieved more often than not by GPs in Great Britain despite their formal undergraduate medical education. Medical education, research and academic medicine in general are based on, and entirely appropriate to, the highly selected clinical material which constitutes the problems of hospital medicine. They remain cut off from the problems of medical care of the GP, operational as well as clinical. Because of the very efficiency of the GP (and other domiciliary care services) they see only those problems which are inappropriate to his form of care or which slip through his preventive and diagnostic system.

Detailed studies (Williamson, Stoke and Gray, 1964) have shown that there may be in general practice a wide range of clinical abnormalities not recorded in the GP's notes. However, Hodgkin (1968) has shown that in his own practice the rates of the conditions known to him and already recorded in his notes are roughly equivalent to the totals unearthed by Williamson *et al.* in their *ad hoc* study. Also many of these conditions, not recorded by the GPs in the Williamson survey, are chronic conditions with no known treatment or where treatment influences the outcome marginally, if at all.

Bearing in mind the criteria proposed by Junger and Wilson for effective presymptomatic and preventive activities, we must beware of diminishing the volume of effective presymptomatic, preventive and, in particular, curative medicine embodied in current conventional general practice, in exchange for time-consuming and relatively unrewarding presymptomatic and preventive procedures.

THE INDIVIDUAL AND THE COMMUNITY

Various problems in this field have been touched on and will not be further developed. They include the general place of, and emphasis on, the individual as an individual *vis-à-vis* the society to which he belongs, as well as the simpler economic considerations. Also included are the more general problems of public health and the social implications of health education in propaganda. For example, what are the relative economic benefits from the following possible mechanisms for reducing smoking: anti-smoking propaganda campaigns in the schools, but also for older age groups; banning all tobacco advertising; and implementing a prohibitive tax?

Studies of the efficacy of medical education deliberately orientated toward specific age groups and at-risk groups in his practice, are being carried out by Dr L. Pike in Birmingham (Pike, 1969). Further studies in this field are urgently needed. These must include a *post hoc* and *procter hoc* measure of the individual patient's knowledge of the particular field to which the propaganda or education is being directed.

COMMUNITY AND HOSPITAL SERVICES

The rational deployment of resources as between the present community and hospital services is prevented partly by lack of real knowledge and partly by the political division of the health services into three main areas: the hospital services on the one hand, and the executive councils and local authority services in the domiciliary field on the other hand. The political issues will be settled by political machinery. However, there are practical implications and difficulties resulting from the separate organisation and loyalties of staff in the three areas when any attempt to build up a 'team' approach is attempted. These will be considered later.

The nodal point of any medical service is the patient with his clinical problem. The deployment of resources to achieve the solution of amelioration of his problem will be a compromise between the economic and administrative needs of centralisation and physical concentration of as much equipment and staff as possible under as few roofs as possible. This concentration is necessary to maximise utilisation of scarce human and physical resources and to minimise the overheads necessary in their deployment. Such concentrations of resources are also necessary for generating a minimal research basis in many fields. The intercommunication problems between separate parts of the system are also reduced, at least at the administrative, if not the clinical, level.

On the other hand, there is a balance between the undoubted savings from concentration of resources and the equally undoubted disadvantages in time spent, inconvenience and cost to the patient of 'over-concentration' geographically, apart from an inevitable loss of the personal element in the clinical situation.

The balance in urban areas seems to be crystallising out at two functional levels. The central, district or area hospital serving a population of up to 500,000 and large enough to supply a wide range of specialist units, on the one hand, and group practice units serving communities of 15,000–20,000 patients on the other hand. In these group practice units would be concentrated all the staff and resources needed for the community services. The community services are mainly concerned with the primary assessment of previously un-differentiated clinical problems, and their subsequent reassessment, the continuing care (or co-ordination of that care) of the chronic sick and physically and mentally disabled of all ages. Such continuing care and co-ordination increasingly involves socio-economic as well as traditional medical services and demands a team approach.

The hospital increasingly concentrates on acute illnesses where diagnostic, nursing and other services, including operative techniques, available only at hospital level are essential. It also has a place in the continuing care of those chronic illnesses occurring infrequently enough for any one GP, even as a therapeutic specialist, to continue to exercise the necessary skills within a population of 20,000 who might attend one group centre.

The Relative Cost of Group Practice and Hospital Buildings and Services

The relative costs of group practice and hospital buildings and services have not yet been evaluated properly or in a wide enough setting and very little can be said about this at the present time. There is considerable information about the cost of a hospital bed and the services that go with the occupancy of such a bed. There is also considerable material available about the capital costs of group practice buildings; and the salaries of the participant health team are either known or can be estimated; but, so far as I know, no real balance sheet has ever been drawn up.

Cost and Effectiveness of Home Care of Serious Illness

The cost and effectiveness of home care of serious illness, on the other hand, has been studied, though once again in a fragmentary way. Crombie (1954) and Crombie and Cross (1959, 1961 and 1963) have looked at the general problem of the home care of serious illness in relation to the care of the same type of illnesses in hospitals.

The findings can be summarised as follows: some 25–40% of the patients in the medical beds of a general hospital have no nursing or technical requirements at a hospital level, other than the need for chest radiography or multiple injections. However, all but $12\frac{1}{2}\%$ were in hospital either because they had no home or no willing and able relative to look after them at home. On very few occasions where a home existed were deficiencies in the structure of the home a bar to home care. The residual $12\frac{1}{2}\%$ who seemed to be in hospital for no identifiable reason of medical, nursing or social deficiency were there for what are best classed as 'reasons of emotional insecurity and inadequacy of the relatives of the sick person'.

Crombie and Cross also showed that for every one of the patients in hospital for no very good nursing or medical reason, there were at least six others with illnesses of equal severity being cared for at home by their GPs. It was also estimated at the time of this study (1954) that home care was costing the family concerned, and the community as a whole, some £6–8 a week, while hospital care would have cost some £30 a week. However, if we remember that for everyone who was costing their own family and the community the smaller sum, there were six of these compared with one in the expensive hospital bed, it can be seen that, in fact, the community would not gain anything by making a *pro rata* payment for the home care of seriously ill patients. The present costs of treating serious illness may be high, but they are being reduced by the hidden subsidy provided by the relatives of those who look after patients with the same serious illnesses in their own homes. We have no reason to believe that a costing at this present time would show a different conclusion in general terms.

Deployment of Diagnostic Services
The deployment of diagnostic services will rationally follow the allocation of the priorities in the assessment processes. Where these favour a primary general assessor, as is taken for granted in the model presented here, then the diagnostic services, where possible, should physically follow the assessors. There is little cost-effectiveness analysis in this field at the present moment, but empirically it would seem that all portable diagnostic equipment could well be distributed peripherally in the group practice centres, where these diagnostic services are used frequently enough in each group practice centre to warrant the cost. For example, it is clear that haemoglobinometers, peak flow meters and, probably, an ECG machine, all qualify for peripheral distribution. It is also probable that even the simplest X-ray machine is too expensive and not used frequently enough to warrant its use outside the hospital setting.

Transport Services for Patients, Records, Specimens
Similar studies will also need to be carried out before we can know whether the services should be transmitted to the patients or, the patients transmitted to the services, and whether the services should be deployed from the peripheral group practice premises or from the central hospital premises. We have done no cost-efficiency studies in this field, though a study of *How Patients Reach the Doctor*

(Hutchinson, 1969) has been carried out by the Research Unit. This was a study in a country town and provides at least a factual basis for further studies of cost efficiency.

The Place of Day Centres

The hospital has an increasingly important place in the deployment of services to the community via centralised day centres where the benefits of centralised, scarce and expensive resources in skilled and specialist manpower, as well as equipment, can be deployed without the additional cost of the patient's hospital care. Such centres are already transforming the care of the mentally ill and of the chronic and aged sick in the community. They could probably transform the care of more long-term problems in paediatrics also, though the present policy of a number of *ad hoc*, highly specialised units for each type of chronic paediatric disability may be the more rational answer to this problem.

Cottage Hospitals, Welfare Homes, Hotel Care Beds in Group Practice Premises (or Welfare-Type Homes)

The place of the cottage hospital seems to have been finally settled on economic grounds. However, we must remember that the cottage hospital bed is simply a down-graded hospital bed and carries all the inevitable inefficiency and inadequacy which such a down-graded service implies in administrative costs alone. There is however, another way of looking at this problem. Many local authorities run welfare homes for the aged where the weekly total cost for the provision of these services, including the servicing of loans and the capital cost of building, etc., is less than £15 a week. Such welfare homes are run by a staff in which the matron and assistant matron are fully qualified nurses and have had administrative nursing experience, at least at the level of a ward sister, while the rest of the staff are recruited, often on a part-time basis, from women who live locally and who have had nursing training in the past. From personal experience of one welfare home in which there are sixty beds, it is clear that such a unit can competently care for serious illnesses of the type we have been describing earlier for up to ten patients at a time without overstressing present staffing. The welfare home bed is, of course, simply an up-graded home bed and not a down-graded hospital bed. I believe that we should explore the possibility of delivering medical care in the community for the type of illness that we have been describing previously from such a welfare home basis. The extra staff to carry the equivalent of sixty ill people, compared with ten, would be, according to estimates made on an *ad hoc* basis, some four full-timers or their equivalent. There would be need for some extra administrative and record staff to carry the increased turnover which would be inevitable. However, the resulting total cost of some £15 per week is very different from the £40+ for the cheapest cottage hospital bed, and I believe the type of care which could be delivered would be in every way comparable in quality. Similar proposals were first made in the Dawson Report.

The Structure of the Domiciliary Health Team in Relation to its Function
The structure of the domiciliary health team to fulfil the functions outlined in the model have been and are the subject of intensive study by many bodies. The Research Unit with the Practice Organisation Committee of the Royal College of General Practitioners have carried out a 'practice activities' study in 100 group practices known to be attempting to use ancillary workers to the full. This study was an attempt to assess not only the present structure of such teams, but also the training which each member of the team had obtained and the job that each member was now fulfilling. One of the most important findings of this study was the non-correlation between past training and present function. It was partly as a result of this that Dr Drury, the recorder for this study, has been involved in setting up, with others, a training programme for medical secretaries. Such programmes are now being run by several Colleges of Further Education and Technology.

Other studies are proceeding on the use of non-medically-qualified personnel as primary clinical assessors. It is too early yet to say how successful, or otherwise, these may be in the situation which obtains in Great Britain today.

Human Relations
The team concept is accepted as inevitable, but there is little application of even the scanty known facts of human relations and group dynamics in the proposals for the structure of such teams.

All human activity is ultimately based on the actions of individuals as individuals or as members of small dynamic groups of six to thirty members. Such groups will be stable and cohesive to the extent that they have: a formal status structure; a set of clearly defined roles, bound together by equally clearly defined interpersonal rules; enough time for respect, regard and liking to result in natural peer bonds between the role-holders; and the sharing of a common world view and set of expectations, attitudes and values.

The incorporation of the maximum of ritualisation in the inter-personal cues and responses, the inclusion of shared orgiastic activities within the formal structure and the presence of outgroups threatening the stability and existence of the group, are all group-strengthening characteristics which, however, cannot, or at least should not, be invoked in the domiciliary health team.

Much work needs to be done on establishing the criteria for stability in group practice and on strengthening the place of the individual as an individual in the professional roles of assessment, rather than on concentrating, as we are now, on sterile demarcation disputes between role-holders. This last exercise seems to be producing an inevitable 'us and them' dichotomy between medically and sociologically trained personnel which stands in good stead for the absence of a threatening out-group.

COMPARATIVE STUDIES OF THE SYSTEM AS A WHOLE

In the end, the only way to establish the credentials of any new proposal is to carry out a trial or pilot study. The only way in which pilot studies of sufficient scope can be mounted is within the structure of a research and development policy on a much larger basis than at present conceived.

The three basic interacting elements in such studies are: first, the group practice with its individual members of the team; second, the district or area hospital; and third, the overall medical care system within which these units and sub-units participate.

The work of the Research Unit and its plans for the future largely consist of intensive studies of the system at the district hospital level and below.

Records

The basis of all such studies must be standardised and adequate record systems. One of the main functions of the Research Unit, from its inception, has been the evolution of such standard recording systems for general practice. They are based on a standardised classification of disease which is, in effect, a short list of the International Classification of Diseases, but appropriate to the conditions of general practice and the relative frequency with which diseases are met in general practice. Record systems, for their full usefulness, require an age/sex register as a base line and these also have been standardised and are described in the appropriate Appendix.

Simple record systems exist for the recording in disease indexes of lists of patients who have suffered from each disease, of patient episode cards in which the set of illnesses suffered by each patient accumulate on a record card appropriate to each patient, and a ledger-sheet-type recording on which the entries are sequential in time. Each system has its appropriate place. The two former have their maximal usefulness in clinical research, while the third is mainly for operational studies. We have also mentioned the Wright paediatric card.

The study of the origin of information used in clinical decision-making is also appropriate to this section and it is from the results of studies of this type that appropriate records systems can be rationally designed.

Information and Communication Systems
In this field the Research Unit has concentrated in the past on the technical problems involved in setting up an integrated information system for medical care. These technical problems were studied in the Stoke project, a study in which an attempt was made to link information about all medical services used by 20,000 patients in the City of Stoke in the twelve months 1964/65. The 20,000 were patients of twelve GPs, and standardised record systems were set up for use by the GPs, the in-patient and out-patient services of the hospitals to which those 20,000 patients might have gone and the forty-odd local authority services who might have provided care for the same group of patients during the twelve-month period. The identification of the patients and linkage of their units from the various contributing services was achieved by a modification of the Hogben number based on part of the patient's surname, Christian name and date of birth. The results of this study are still being analysed. This study was also concerned with an assessment of the ways in which people of different

sex, age and social status might use different parts of the health care and local authority services.

The evaluation of the usefulness of such an integrated information system is best considered under three separate headings: clinical, research and administrative payoffs. The research potential and the administrative payoffs from such integrated record systems are already evident. However, it is still very unclear what the payoff for clinical purposes will be. The study on the origin of information used in clinical decision-making makes it clear that we should be careful not to assume that there is an automatic payoff in this field.

Recommendations

The organisational problem involved in setting up the trials and studies necessary quickly and economically to settle the most effective types of medical care systems, are such that they can only be carried out by some large centralised body with large funds. A Medical Care Development Corporation is required which would absorb the present Department of Health Working Parties on Record Systems etc. A wide range of studies should be undertaken; e.g. one study must be large enough to test the Area Health Board concept, another the various formulations of personnel and other resources at the *smallest* unit of any new system, namely the district or sector hospital and its associated domiciliary services.

The setting up of such a centralised corporation would not preclude the present *ad hoc* approach by interested bodies and individuals. On the other hand, this latter activity is an essential complement to any centralised planning.

These surveys are so important for future medical care and the NHS that they must be prosecuted with vigour and on a sufficiently large scale.

Ad Hoc *Studies*

These studies of the system as a whole have already been mentioned. They include the Harborne/Castle Vale experiment and the development of an integrated group practice/district hospital information system.

The research unit is also engaged in a preliminary study of the attitudes and values of the participants in the group practice team, as well as an evaluation of the more objectively measurable characteristics of such groups. We believe that this is an important and largely neglected field. There are obvious difficulties and work is at a very preliminary stage.

Research Methodology

The Research Unit of the Royal College of General Practitioners is basically an advisory service to GPs as individuals, or groups, in the fields of clinical, epidemiological and operational research. The tools of this research are records, primarily, but the main function of the Research Unit is, in fact, to help such practitioners to identify clearly their problem and then to assist them in setting up a rational problem-solving situation. We believe that this is, in fact, our major contribution to research in medical care, rather than any specific projects of our own which we may have completed, initiated or may carry out in the future.

Appendix 1

CO-ORDINATED RESEARCH AND DEVELOPMENT IN THE NATIONAL HEALTH SERVICE

AN INSTITUTE OF COMMUNITY CARE I

The NHS, with its centrally administered, even if tripartite structure, provides unique opportunities for the study and trial of new systems of integrated medical care. The opportunities for this creative integration are provided by the sophisticated techniques of data-processing as the basis for more powerful information systems and organisation and method, and systems analysis in the development of more powerful organisational and control systems.

Evolution of Medical Care

The main components of any medical care system are the resources based centrally in hospitals and those based peripherally in the domiciliary field. The greatest immediate returns in terms of an enhanced quality of medical service with maximum use of all resources—staff (medically-qualified and non-medically-qualified), buildings, fixed equipment, mobile equipment and capital—will come from employing systems which integrate, wherever possible the presently separated components. (In this, local authority resources are included in the domiciliary field.)

The long-term improvements will come from re-examining the traditional roles of the present participants and the system in which they operate, by setting up trial situations where the staff and other resources are deployed on an integrated basis (see memo on midwifery services for example and the McKeown concept of the team of clinicians to replace the present generalist).

The most important long-term organisational problem is to establish the constitution of the medical care team. In particular the deployment of medically-qualified *vis-à-vis* non-medically-qualified staff of various types; and generalists *vis-à-vis* specialists in the domiciliary field of health care.

In parallel with the re-examination of traditional roles will go the development of an integrated information system based on a records system centralised, probably, on the sector or district hospital computer. The organisational problem in the management of this new complex will have to be examined *pari passu*.

The creative interaction of these three main lines of approach will provide new ideas for trial, and an overriding consideration in any such study of the integration of medical care agencies, must be a system which puts a premium on the organisation of such exploratory pilot studies and trials of all kinds.

The immediate integration of the record systems for a $7\frac{1}{2}\%$ sample sector hospital area population with that of the sector hospital, is the subject of a separate memorandum.

The Place of the Institute

The institute responsible for this development programme must obviously involve staff from all branches of present medical care, including the specialised units such as social medicine, operational research and hospital management, if it is to fulfil its main evolutionary function.

This unit will also need a sufficient operational background if the results are to be significant; the minimum size would seem to be a hospital unit of the size of the present sector or district hospital with its sector population of some 130,000 people. The unit would not itself be concerned directly with the clinical care of patients.

Subsidiary Functions

The Institute of Community Care would also be a clearing house for other activities involving both the domiciliary and hospital components. For example, there would be unique opportunities: for the continuing study of the natural history of the self-limiting but non-lethal commoner diseases, of the chronic and degenerative diseases and of the epidemiology of these diseases; for studies based on representative samples of the population; for the evaluation of various prophylactic techniques; for the teaching, both undergraduate and postgraduate, of these matters; and for the integration with other disciplines such as sociology and social geography which would have access to the same defined population.

The domiciliary field would enable the setting up of various types of model practices, and would also provide educational opportunities, not only in the research and organisational techniques themselves but also in the practical application of research. It is at this point in the scheme that the Research Advisory Service of the College (the subject of a separate memorandum (B)) would have its place.

It would also provide a nodal point for symposia and discussions concerning the future work of the Research Unit and of the practical implications of completed work.

Summary
The main opportunities for such an institute are operational and clinical. The situation is creative in that the possibilities cannot all be anticipated and will only emerge as a result of the interactions which will deliberately take place.

The Institute will have a continuing function in that it will be the nodal point for exploring the impact of new ideas and techniques, both operational and clinical, on the traditional pattern of medical care at the sector hospital level of the system. There is of course a place for similar institutes to explore the situation at other levels in the system.

One institute as proposed would be unlikely to cope with all the organisational and clinical problems at the sector hospital level as outlined, so there will almost certainly be a need for others whose activities will need to be centrally co-ordinated. Also there will be need for similar 'research and development' units at all other levels in the NHS, particularly at the level of the basic domiciliary care unit in 'model practices', which may or may not resemble present group practice, and also at the level of the Area Health Board or its equivalent.

The central co-ordination of these activities will demand a department of 'research and development' within the framework of the NHS.

AN INSTITUTE OF COMMUNITY CARE II

Integration of Domiciliary and Hospital Records
The Institute of Community Care would co-ordinate the research

projects conducted within the sector hospital operational area. This would include projects involving patients residing in the sector hospital area whether treated at home or in the sector hospital beds. It should also include medical care from all other sources and would therefore include the local authority services.

The basis of this co-ordinated research, whose ultimate aim is an integrated medical care system, would be an information system based on the linkage of all records, from whatever source, concerning the services given and/or required by each individual in the sector hospital area community (population 130,000±).

The Opportunities

The opportunities presented by general practice are unique because 80–90% of all illness treated by doctors in the community is dealt with entirely by GPs without referral for consultant or specialist opinion. Also, the GP is the only member of the health team in a position to co-ordinate or monitor the activities of all other members of the team.

The College Records Unit

The Records Unit of the College of General Practitioners with the College Research Adviser, has evolved record systems for use in general practice which can be used for such a linkage system.

Current Systems

The Records and Statistics Unit, accommodated in the Birmingham Regional Hospital Board headquarter offices, has co-ordinated numerous teams of GP recorders using the standardised systems developed by the Unit. The information is recorded either in a disease index, on patient summary cards (age/sex register cards) or in a day ledger. The data recorded are pre-coded and capable of direct transfer to punch cards or magnetic tape. Material collected by one method is directly comparable with that collected by the others. In all systems the following information is recorded for each episode of illness:

(a) the date of consultation,
(b) the patient's surname and forenames,
(c) the patient's date of birth, sex, marital status and social status,

(d) the diagnosis, and

(e) the doctor's code number.

(The first three letters of the surname, the first letter of the first forename, the full date of birth of the patient and the code number of the patient's doctor are used for record identification and linkage purposes.)

All record systems have space for additional *ad hoc* information, but even the recording in these sections, e.g. for referrals, is systematised as far as possible. A compendium of codes is being prepared.

The number of practitioners using these standardised systems has increased from the original twelve doctors, who have kept continuous records for the past six years, to a total of over one hundred now.

Current Analyses

The records can be abstracted annually, to yield information about the workload of each GP and of the illnesses for which his patients attend him. Abstractions at weekly intervals concerning infections and communicable illnesses are carried out and co-ordinated with clinico-pathological and bacteriological data at the Central Public Health Service Laboratory at Colindale. These latter analyses are based on disease indexes kept by some sixty GPs—caring for 150,000 people, a representative sample of the general population.

The more long-term projects of the Records and Statistics Unit would be concerned with:

(a) linkage of information about care provided by other medical agencies for the patients in the recording practices;

(b) the positive and negative associations of morbidity during the lifetime of individuals; and

(c) the association of measurable environmental features with the observed morbidity pattern.

The opportunities for linkage studies on a large scale have been explored in a pilot study carried out for twelve months during 1964/65, in twelve practices in the City of Stoke involving 25,000 people, a representative sample of the population. The analysis of this material presents certain problems which can be handled only by computers. The results of this study should lead the way to more comprehensive linkage studies.

The preliminary study of patterns of association of illnesses will be explored by an analysis of the accumulated five years' recorded data from the twelve practitioners who constituted the original Records Unit Working Party and who will, we hope, continue this recording indefinitely. Preliminary studies of the technical problems involved in this would be carried out on the material accumulated during the past five years by Dr H. W. K. Acheson (a member of the Working Party), GP in Stoke.

Other problems involving sophisticated data-processing techniques have been explored by the Records Unit Working Party. For example, Dr James Scott, medical officer to the students at Keele University, has with Mr I. Cooper, of the Department of Theoretical Physics and Chemistry, prepared a computer programme for the conversion of data in disease index form into patient summary card form and vice versa. This programme also carried out other analyses, such as incidence rates for morbidity, at the same time.

The Sector Hospital Information System

Phase I. The system of general practice recording described above has been used for the past six years by one practice in the sector hospital area whose patients represent a $7\frac{1}{2}\%$ ± sample of its population. This information is available now for computer input since the same linkage system has been used as that adopted by the sector hospital record system and would constitute *Phase I* of the linkage operation.

Phase II. There are opportunities for recording additional standardised information which might be considered useful for this next phase of the linkage project. For example: referrals for consultant opinion, clinical pathology, radiography and other services, whether to the sector hospital or other hospitals; treatment given; services given by others in the domiciliary field, e.g. local authority workers (DN, MW, HH, SW, HV, MHV, etc.); and additional social data, e.g. home conditions and facilities for domiciliary care of serious illness. Codes have already been devised for many of these.

Phase III. The next phase of the linkage project would involve the recording of data whose value would only become evident during the second phase. This would include selective feedback of hospital-derived data to the domiciliary field.

Phase IV would involve extension of systems to the other practices in the sector hospital area.

The evolution of more effective information systems for medical care will be created by the opportunities provided by the first three phases of recording, and also by the integration which will follow the interaction between the presently separated departments of medical care which even simple record linkage will make possible.

The full benefits of such integration of records to the participants in medical care who use them can only be made evident by deliberately setting up a creative situation of the type embodied in this memorandum.

AN INSTITUTE OF COMMUNITY CARE III

Research Practice for the Study of Surveillance and Pre-symptomatic Diagnosis Techniques

The practice of medicine has traditionally been concerned with cure but has now also to deal with prevention of disease. The study of the latter has taken place in relative isolation from the former and the practised integration of preventive with curative medicine is an urgent necessity.

Knowledge of preventive techniques in the field of carcinoma of the cervix and breast, diabetes, glaucoma, phenylketonuria, obesity, alcoholism, rhesus incompatibility, hypertension, chronic urinary infection, to name only the most obvious, is growing rapidly at the level of understanding of the natural history of the conditions concerned and the theoretical complications of presymptomatic diagnosis and prevention. This memorandum concerns one suggestion for evaluating the practical implementation of the results of such research while providing a basis for further research studies at the same time.

In this country the role of assessor of previously undiagnosed clinical conditions is almost entirely filled by the GP and it is at this point in the chain of medical care that presymptomatic diagnosis and prevention must be primarily applied.

The other more theoretical role of the GP concerns personal doctoring, and to the extent that he is the main co-ordinator of the other sources of medical care, he must also be the point at which surveillance efforts should be primarily concentrated.

If this preliminary assessment is valid then it follows that we should be urgently concerned with exploration of the ways in which the new knowledge about preventable disease could be exploited via general practice. The proposal is that this should be done by setting up certain general practice research units. The form of these units will be dictated by the problems requiring solution.

The Important Problems
1. Continuing study of the natural history of disease and the establishment of normal values as a base line to all other studies.
2. Establishing what conditions can be prevented or mitigated by early diagnosis.
3. Establishing ever more economic methods for uncovering preventable diseases.
4. Establishing ever more effective mechanisms for preventing or mitigating diseases of all sorts.
5. Integrating the results of the above research in clinical medical practice. Since these will be frequently changing and extending in scope, this will demand a dynamic approach with little hope of any once-for-all type of organisational answer.

Dealing with the Problems
As in all problem-solving, an approach based on the maximum of specialisation on detail with the maximum of integration of results at all levels is most likely to produce a satisfactory solution. It is obvious that the former element of specialisation can be dealt with by special units set up to study *ad hoc* problems (e.g. the MRC Unit in South Wales *par excellence* but also the Birmingham and Bedford Diabetes Working Parties).

However the only way in which the broader picture can be obtained is from a defined representative population studied in depth, once again as by the MRC Unit in South Wales, but there is also a place for units which will concentrate on the wider ramifications of the natural history of disease. The College of General Practitioners already have an organised network of GPs who keep morbidity records in a standardised disease index in which information can accumulate over the years. The main purpose of accumulating this data is to study the negative and positive correlation between specific diseases in one individual over years; to provide a base line for the incidence and prevalence of definable disease conditions on a continuing basis and as a supplement to this, weekly returns of communicable and infectious diseases; to provide a source of data for retrospective studies (e.g. on the relationship of thrombo-embolic disorders and oral contraceptives).

Apart from this there are individual units concentrating on other special aspects of morbidity, e.g. the familial incidence of common and uncommon diseases.

Such basic data will be essential for the evaluation of surveillance and presymptomatic diagnostic techniques. Practices of this type form a ready made basis for the implementation immediately of such organisational studies.

The requirements for such research practices would be an element of medical and secretarial overstaffing and the attachment from time to time on an *ad hoc* basis, of paramedical and ancillary workers.

OBJECTIVES AND ACTIVITIES OF THE RESEARCH UNIT OF THE ROYAL COLLEGE OF GENERAL PRACTITIONERS

The objectives are:

I. (a) to provide a source of advice based on increasing experience for GPs and medical or other specialists;

(b) to provide a service to GPs and other workers by collection and handling of data;

(c) to initiate and carry out epidemiological and operational research projects.

II. The implementation of these objectives has involved:

(a) discussion of the aims and objectives of research studies;

(b) consideration of methods appropriate to the achievement of these aims;

(c) the design of suitable records and methods for their use in practice;

(d) reference to other appropriate sources of advice sometimes suggested, whether clinical, organisational or specialised, beyond the College's own resources;

(e) advice on costing of the various processes included in a research project;

(f) assistance with the analysis of results, especially where punch card or computer equipment was required;

(g) the preparation of tabulations and their interpretation;

(h) the preparation of conclusions for publication.

III. The service undertakes the design and testing of new record systems for clinical, epidemiological and organisational research in general practice.

IV. The service maintains contact with others whose work, actively or potentially, coincide with its own. These contacts include individuals, outside bodies and other committees of the College.

V. The service, through its standardised systems of recording, provides a basis for the continuous assessment of the work of GPs in both epidemiological and operational senses. Within this framework special studies of particular problems are planned and undertaken at will.

VI. The service has for some time operated a system by which periodic returns are made by a network of field observers in general practice. For the time being, weekly returns of communicable diseases, specified accidents and certain other conditions are analysed and made available to others inside and outside the College.

VII. The service initiates and executes *ad hoc* epidemiological and operational studies which make use of the information collected by members of its observer network.

VIII. The service provides other workers in the research field of general practice with access to records kept in standardised fashion.

IX. The service organises special studies on behalf of the Research Committee and other Committees of Council of the College.

X. The service undertook studies of fundamental principles applied in medical practice, as, for example, studies of the diagnostic process and the enumeration of diagnostic data at presymptomatic and symptomatic levels.

XI. The service also studies the association between data relating to morbidity and data concerning features of the environment.

REFERENCES

Crombie, D. L., *An Assessment of Medical Care*, Thesis, Birmingham University, 1954.

Crombie, D. L. (a) 'The Defects of General Practice', *Lancet*, vol. 1, 1963, p. 209.

Crombie, D. L. (b) 'The Procrustean Bed of Medical Nomenclature', *Lancet*, vol. 1, 1963, p. 1205.

Crombie, D. L. (c) 'Diagnostic Process', *J. Coll. Gen. Pract.*, vol. 6, 1963, p. 579.

Crombie, D. L. (d) 'Diagnostic Methods', *Practitioner*, vol. 191, 1963, p. 539.

Crombie, D. L., 'Testing in Family for Diabetes', *J. Coll. Gen. Pract.*, vol. 7, 1964, p. 379.

Crombie, D. L., 'Preventive Medicine and Presymptomatic Diagnosis', *J. Coll. Gen. Pract.*, vol. 15, 1968, p. 344.

Crombie, D. L., and Cross, K. W., 'The Contribution of the Nurse in General Practice', *Brit. J. of Prev. and Soc. Med.*, vol. 11, 1957, p. 41.

Crombie, D. L., and Cross, K. W., 'Serious Illness in Hospital and at Home', *Medical Press*, vol. CCXLII, 1959, p. 6284.

Crombie, D. L., and Cross, K. W., 'The Care of Seriously Ill Patients in Hospital and General Practice', *J. Coll. Gen. Pract.*, vol. 14, 1961, p. 270.

Crombie, D. L., and Cross, K. W., 'The Relationship of Hospital and Domiciliary Care', *Medical Care*, vol. 1, 1963, p. 245.

Crombie, D. L., and Cross, K. W., 'The Work load in General Practice', *Lancet*, vol. 2, 1964, p. 354.

Hodgkin, K., and Gillie, C., 'Relieving the Strain by Work Study and a Practice Nurse in a Two-Doctor Urban Practice', In: Royal College of General Practitioners, *The Practice Nurse*, Reports from General Practice, No. 10, London 1968.

Horder, J., and Horder E., 'Illness in General Practice', *The Practitioner*, vol. 173, 1954, p. 177.

Hutchinson, M., 'How Patients get to the Surgery', *J. Coll. Gen. Pract.*, vol. 18, 1969, p. 95.

Logan, W. P. D., *G.R.O. Studies on Medical and Population Subjects*, No. 7, London 1953 (H.M.S.O.).

Logan, W. P. D., *G.R.O. Studies on Medical and Population Subjects*, No. 9, London 1956 (H.M.S.O.).

Logan, W. P. D., and Cushion, A. A., (a) *G.R.O. Studies on Medical and Population Subjects*, No. 14, London 1958 (H.M.S.O.).

Logan, W. P. D., and Cushion, A. A., (b) *A National Morbidity Survey*, General Register Officer, vols 1–3, London 1958 (H.M.S.O.).

McKeown, T., 'The British National Health Service in Perspective', *Journal of Hygiene*, vol. 17, 1963, p. 233.

Morris, J. N., Kegan, A., and Pattison, D. C., 'Incidence and Prediction of Ischaemic Heart-disease in London Busmen', *Lancet*, vol. 2, 1966, p. 553.

Pike, L. A., 'A Screening Programme for the Elderly in General Practice', *The Practitioner*, vol. 203, 1969, p. 805.

Royal College of General Practitioners, 'Diabetes Survey Working Party', *British Medical Journal*, vol. 1, 1962, p. 1497.

Royal College of General Practitioners, 'Diabetes Survey Working Party', *British Medical Journal*, vol. 2, 1963, p. 655.

Royal Society of Medicine, 'Symposium on Presymptomatic Diagnosis', *Proceedings*, vol. 59, No. 11, 1966.

D

Ryle, A., 'The Neurosis in a General Practice Population', *J. Coll. Gen. Pract.*, vol. 3, 1960, p. 313.

Williamson, J., Stoke, I. H., Gray, S., *et al.*, 'Old People at Home: their Unreported Needs', *Lancet*, vol. 1, 1964, p. 1117.

Wilson, J. M. G., and Jungfer, G., *Principles and Practice of Screening for Diseases*, WHO Information Publication, Geneva 1967.

COMMENT ON 'A MODEL OF THE MEDICAL CARE SYSTEM: A GENERAL SYSTEMS APPROACH'

J. M. G. WILSON

Department of Health and Social Security

Crombie, writing from the family doctor's viewpoint, bases his economic commentary on general practice and the current developments of primary medical care in relation to hospital and community care. He points to the considerable difficulties in arriving at answers to the question of the best and most economical provision of medical care in the absence of certain basic knowledge. Great importance is rightly given to the need for an information system that can give ready access to data that has been collected in a standardised way. On pp. 65–76 of his paper Crombie contrasts two kinds of information systems. In one, the conventional kind, much factual data is accumulated about patients, a great deal of which will not be relevant to future situations and hence will not be needed again. The other type of information is what the author terms 'nodal', by which he means information terms which carry with them a wealth of connotations about social and medical factors in the lives of patients (e.g. 'drinks too much' or 'dirty house'). There is surely room for error here in that information systems need to use terms with carefully defined meanings which carry the same message to each user; and it is just the difficulty in breaking down the highly connotative terms used by doctors (form of medical shorthand) which constitutes an obstacle to the development of generally useful medical information systems.

Some emphasis has been given to the above remarks because they seem to epitomise the author's strongly held view that the GP, as the continuing medical adviser of his patients, offers greater value in the primary assessment (or diagnosis) of illness than other providers of medical care, e.g. specialists. The argument is that the one adviser accumulates over the years of his practice an unrivalled knowledge of the social and medical histories of his patients, a knowledge that specialists could not attain unless they became generalists as well. The value of making the comparison is agreed and Crombie cites the trial to be conducted in Birmingham of comparing traditional group general practice with general practice in a health centre, the medical staff of which are specialised in it, training as obstetrician, paediatrician and geriatric physician. In a comparison of this kind perhaps the greatest difficulty is likely to be the measurement of output, in this case the result of the two different kinds of medical care. It should be relatively easy to measure such variables as the use of services, the amount of morbidity and mortality, and the loss of working time in sickness absence; but to date there are no effective methods of measuring the progress and severity of different disease processes and their effect on the life of the patient. It will be interesting to see the way in which these problems are handled in the trial.

Crombie includes presymptomatic diagnosis in his model of medical care, which raises yet more severe difficulties in assessing what has been achieved in economic terms. One of the chief reasons is that, as yet, we are dealing with even softer data in the realm of diagnosis and treatment before the appearance of well-defined clinical disease. Crombie rightly pleads for elucidation of the problems by epidemiological surveys before large-scale screening programmes are begun. In this context the author has played a leading part in the long-term evaluation of screening for early diabetes mellitus in Birmingham. He has come to the firm conclusion that a general screening programme for all age groups is not justified and that, for economic as well as other reasons, an attack on particular high-risk groups of people, carried out as part of the routine medical services rather than as an *ad hoc* programme, is the best approach. This is much in keeping with the views of other workers in this field.

After discussing the role of the primary provider of medical care, Crombie turns to the setting in which it is provided, and discusses community and hospital services. Research by himself and Cross has shown that only about 12% of patients actually needed to be in hospital because of the technical facilities there that could not be provided more cheaply and conveniently elsewhere. He does, however, point out that community care is at least in part cheaper because nursing and other care is absorbed by the patient's family circle and that, economically, like has not been compared with like. This is an important point, not so far put to the test, that domiciliary care is assumed to be cheaper than hospital care. Clearly, hospital care needs to be compared, as Reid and Cochrane among others have pointed out, with a similar level of care in the community. Trials along these lines are badly needed. The comparison between hospital intensive care and home care for patients with acute myocardial infarction (heart attacks) in the West Country (carried out by Mather and his colleagues) is along these lines, but there home care does not provide the same facilities as hospital care—a different hypothesis is being tested: 'do patients with acute myocardial infarction do equally well at home as in a hospital intensive care unit?'; not: 'what is the cost of providing the same care in hospital and home?'.

Crombie discusses what degree of diagnostic and other facilities can most economically be provided in group practices and health centres. He takes the size of a group practice to be about 20,000 people and bases his argument on that population. However, there are many other factors to be considered than diagnostic facilities. The first question to be decided is surely the best size of the practice, taking into account geography, dispersal of the population, methods of transport, etc. The question of equipment, particularly X-ray equipment, is being looked at by the Scottish Home and Health Department, which is studying their use in health centres of different size and geographical location.

Lastly, Crombie rules out the 'cottage hospital' on economic grounds. It has certainly been the policy of the Department of Health and Social Security to close uneconomic hospitals, which has frequently meant small hospitals. However, it is recognised that there may well be room, particularly in country areas, for a type of hospital care intermediate between the large district general hospital and the health centre, where beds can be provided for patients needing some hospital care (e.g. geriatric) not at the level of the district general hospital and nearer to the patients' immediate community. The need for this 'community hospital' is being looked at in the Oxford Hospital Region. The idea is of considerable economic interest since a survey must look at the whole relationship between hospital and community services *vis-à-vis* their efficiency, effectiveness and cost. It is interesting that Crombie makes the comparison between hospital and welfare home costs (£15 a week for the welfare home compared with over £40 for hospital care) and suggests exploring the possibility of using welfare homes for the admission of mentally ill, chronically sick and aged patients. While McKeown would have all these hospital facilities in the one focus there is more to be said, surely, for developing these community hospitals (if they prove to be medically, socially and economically viable) in areas where access to the district general hospital is difficult because of distance.

Chapter III

ECONOMIC ANALYSIS AS A MEANS OF PROGRAMME ASSESSMENT

THE ECONOMICS OF MASS RADIOGRAPHY[1]

J. D. POLE

University College of South Wales and Monmouthshire, Cardiff

'We need to know when to give up mass radiography. One approach to this problem is the purely economic one. Screening should be given up when it costs more to diagnose a case than not to diagnose a case. The present cost of diagnosis is known, but the cost of not diagnosing a case is difficult to calculate accurately.'[2]

THE ECONOMICS OF SCREENING PROGRAMMES

There were two main objects in attempting this study: firstly, to try to articulate the economic analyses adduced by the proponents and critics of screening programmes;[3] secondly, to apply them to a specific disease if possible. Pulmonary tuberculosis was chosen for the latter exercise, as the screenable disease for which the data appeared likely to be the most abundant and reliable, to see how far an economic appraisal could go in the most favourable circumstances. It has not been possible yet to produce quantitative results, and this paper confines itself to setting out the problem and discussing some of the areas of difficulty.

Epidemiologists and public health administrators concerned with what may perhaps be called macro-medical phenomena must always have been aware of economic aspects of their work. Control and eradication programmes for endemic diseases, particularly in poor

---

[1] This paper is based on a study supported by the Nuffield Provincial Hospitals Trust. It has benefited from the comments not only of participants in the symposium but also of Drs J. Meijer and K. Styblo of KNCV, The Hague. Remaining errors are the responsibility of the author.

[2] A. L. Cochrane and V. Springett in: T. McKeown (ed.), *Screening in Medical Care*, The Nuffield Provincial Hospitals Trust, London 1969, p. 121 (O.U.P.).

[3] Screening tests are meant rapidly to sort out apparently well persons who probably have a disease from those who probably do not. Cf. J. M. G. Wilson and G. Jungner, *The Principles and Practice of Screening for Disease*, W.H.O. Technical Report 34, Geneva 1966, p. 11.

countries, must always have been constrained by resource limitations in quite obvious ways, which would inevitably lead to some appraisal of their cost-effectiveness. The reasons can be found both in the large-scale nature of the work and in the public sources from which it has to be financed.

Recently there has been a great increase in interest in such methods, and particularly in mass screening programmes. This interest is focussed however on areas of disease control lying outside the traditional public health sector. The resource implications of these methods, whether in terms of finance or of medical and paramedical manpower are potentially very large, and they can hardly be put into effect without some degree of economic evaluation.

Screening programmes may have various objectives:

1. In the case of communicable diseases, it is a possible *public health measure*, capable of reducing the incidence of the disease in the population by isolating or curing cases at an early stage before they can transmit the disease.

Screening may be preferred to mass prophylaxis in such a situation on the grounds of cost or possible harmful effects of prophylaxis. There is in fact a method of prophylaxis against TB in widespread use, namely BCG vaccination, usually following a tuberculin test.

2. Early diagnosis may *improve the prognosis* for the cases found. In cancers, for instance, it seems to be important to treat the disease, if possible, before it starts to spread about the body.

Most of the screening programmes now being put into operation or discussed have this second objective as their main one. In fact, much of the recent increase in interest in screening techniques arises from the changed epidemiological situation in which the prevalence has increased of non-infectious diseases which are insidious in their onset and unresponsive to ordinary methods of treatment. Mass miniature radiography (MMR) is untypical therefore in this respect, because the prevention of the transmission of the disease has always been regarded medically as the major objective, although from the point of view of the individual member of the public the effect on prognosis probably carries more weight in most cases nowadays. It thus provides an instance of the economic distinction between internal and external economies, to the extent of having the character of either a private or a public good, according to emphasis.

3. It has been strongly argued by some proponents of screening

that it may well be a *cost-saving device*, generally or in specific cases. At first sight, a substantial part of any benefits from MMR could well take this form, either by reducing the cost of treating the particular cases diagnosed, or by the avoidance of the costs of treating secondary cases.

However, one of the difficulties about MMR is that it is rather unspecific in terms of infectious cases found, and also reveals a large number of miscellaneous tuberculous and non-tuberculous abnormalities. Many of these demand treatment or supervision, often with small prospects of significantly improving the prognosis, so that, for instance, poor countries with small health budgets may be saddled with large numbers of low priority cases by the use of MMR,[4] while in richer countries there is a high yield of carcinomas, for which the prognosis is poor.

4. Screening techniques have been advocated as a means of *economising the use of doctors' time*, as they generally make less intensive direct use of medical manpower than non-screening methods of diagnosis. It is too easily assumed that this is necessarily a point in favour. If it were the case that the ratio of marginal productivity to earnings is greater for medical than for the substitutable factors this would be so, but there is a lack of clear evidence to this effect. It is not sufficient to point to the 'shortage' of doctors to demonstrate it.[5]

5. There are some *economies of scale* attaching to screening, which are mutually related,[6] such as:

(a) the use of 'multiphasic' screening, in which a number of tests are applied at the same examination. There are evidently strong elements of 'jointness' between tests which use blood samples, for example, and there are obvious indivisibilities relating to administrative procedures, patients' time, etc., and

(b) the development of automatic processing devices, which operate at rapid speeds and perform a number of analyses on a single small sample.

[4] M. S. Feldstein, 'Health Sector Planning in Developing Countries', *Economica* N.S., vol. XXXVII, No. 146, May 1970, pp. 139–63.

[5] D. E. Yett, 'Causes and Consequences of Salary Differentials in Nursing', *Inquiry*, vol. VII, No. 1, March 1970, pp. 78–99.

[6] T. W. Weber and A. W. Schoen, 'Problems and Trends in Health Evaluation and Screening Procedures', in: W. Hobson (ed.), *The Theory and Practice of Public Health*, 3rd ed., London 1969 (O.U.P.).

6. *Distributional considerations* are emphasised by some proponents of screening methods. There is some evidence that the extent of use even of free health services is directly related to income, either as a consequence of differences in level of health education or of different cultural patterns and attitudes, or for some other reason. More significantly, in many cases the prevalence of disease is greater among the lower income and social groups. Screening is therefore seen as a form of, or substitute for, health education, partly with the aim of improving the income-wise distribution of health services. As such, it must be compared with more direct forms of health education. However, response rates to screening programmes tend to show an even stronger correlation with class and income, notably for some diseases, such as cervical cancer, which are inversely so correlated in their incidence. As a case in point, the possibility has been suggested that 'mass radiography should be confined to groups with high prevalence rates of pulmonary tuberculosis—elderly males, alcoholics, vagrants, etc.—but none of these are easy to drive into the MMR fold.'[7]

7. There is evidence of a considerable mass of *undiagnosed, untreated disease* in the population which may never come to light.[8] This is the mass of the 'clinical iceberg'. How far it is possible and desirable to identify this disease through screening is a complex question which certainly has economic implications.[9]

MASS MINIATURE RADIOGRAPHY: THE COSTS

A trivial ambiguity complicates the discussion of costs in health services. Medicine is not generally aimed at making the patient preternaturally healthy, but at preventing a loss of health. Illness itself therefore has 'costs', which medicine is designed to prevent.

In an ideal world it would be desirable to 'compare the costs of screening with those of not screening' in the sense of simply finding out which were larger in terms of a simple money measure. This would be the relevant exercise in attempting to allocate an optimal health budget. In considering the actual situation, however, it is

[7] A. L. Cochrane and C. M. Fletcher, *The Early Diagnosis of Some Diseases of the Lung*, Office of Health Economics, London 1968.

[8] Cf. W. J. H. Butterfield, *Priorities in Medicine*, The Nuffield Provincial Hospitals Trust, London 1968, Ch. 2 (O.U.P.).

[9] Cf. M. S. Feldstein, *loc. cit.*

rather a question of making the best use of a given quantity of health resources. It is therefore necessary to distinguish between those 'costs' which impinge on the health service budget and those which do not.

The aggregate cost of the Mass Radiography Services is only a little over £1 million per annum, and is thus little more than 0·05% of the total NHS expenditure. The cost has declined slightly in real terms over the past ten years, apparently as a result of some contraction in the service.

The official returns report the cost per 100 examinations for each radiography unit broken down into a number of cost categories. The extraordinary variations in the costs of different units, not only for total costs per 100 examinations but for the major components, suggest either that there are major variations in efficiency or that the accounting conventions used are lacking in uniformity. Economies of scale may be a factor, but these are not detectable by a comparison of population densities of areas covered. Overall, the cost per 100 persons examined was a little over £30.

More important than cost per person or per 100 persons examined is the cost per case found. The statistics distinguish between 'active' and 'other' cases of TB, and between TB and other abnormalities. The cost per 'active' case found varies from about £250 for some units to over £3,000 for others, showing an approximately exponential relation to cases found per 100 examinations. The average cost per active case found in 1967/68 was £414 for mobile units and £323 for static units.

The cost per 100 persons examined was slightly higher, however, for static than for mobile units. The difference reflects the higher proportion of cases found by static units, because static units examine a higher proportion of persons referred by doctors, mainly as contacts. To this extent the static units understate the cost of the service as a true screening procedure, as the term denotes the absence of particular grounds for referral. Short of total eradication, there will always be a need for referral facilities, and the cost-effectiveness of miniature radiography should certainly be considered from this point of view also.

Historically in Britain, and currently in poor countries, pulmonary TB is one of the most important diseases. Its economic importance is increased by the fact that a considerable proportion of its victims are young adults. There has, however, been a strong downward trend in the incidence and prevalence of TB in Britain and other advanced countries over the past 100 years. As a consequence of the fall in prevalence the real cost of finding a case of TB has been rising rapidly. Immigration from high-prevalence countries has clouded the picture somewhat but if the previous trends continue there will come a time when mass radiography is obviously unreasonably expensive. The prospect is of an increase in cost per case found of some 60% over five years. Given the trend, one could set a maximum acceptable average cost per case found and then predict the time at which screening should be abandoned. The existence of this trend, while it adds a certain interest and even topicality to the economic issue, evidently complicates the epidemiological picture at any particular time.

Apart from the direct costs of radiography and of diagnostic follow-up of positives, it is necessary to consider also the costs of treatment, which enter into a discussion of MMR in three ways:

1. Early diagnosis will cause a number of people to be treated who would otherwise have healed naturally. It will also cause others, possibly a large number, to be supervised without treatment, who would not otherwise have imposed this cost.
2. It may reduce the cost of treating those who would otherwise have been treated at a later stage. How far this is so is partly a technical and partly an administrative question.
3. It will totally avoid the cost of treating those who would become infected and be treated as a result of the original cases not having been diagnosed, isolated and rendered inactive.

The costs of treating an active case found by screening do not appear to differ materially from those of treating symptomatic cases. Any such differences are, in any event, small by comparison with those between the costs of hospital and domiciliary treatment respectively. A curious feature of the hospital treatment of pulmonary tuberculosis is that in the majority of cases its therapeutic value is largely restricted to monitoring potentially unco-operative patients. There are two main reasons for non-co-operation: the rapidity with which drugs operate to stop tuberculous activity and the disagreeable aspects of the drugs themselves. The cost-effectiveness of individual drugs in this sense should be considered.

THE BENEFITS

The central problem in assessing the cost-effectiveness of a screening programme is to identify the medical gains resulting from presumptive earlier diagnosis. So far as their significance for MMR is concerned, the relevant questions are:

1. How far in advance of symptomatic diagnosis, in terms of time, and of the development of the disease, would MMR have been likely to pick up the case?
2. How would any difference in the condition of the patient at diagnosis have affected (a) morbidity, (b) mortality or (c) disability?
3. What difference would the earlier diagnosis and isolation have made to the probability of other persons becoming infected with the disease?

The decline in the incidence of the disease, which has given rise to the increase in cost per case found, appears to be largely independent of an even more striking phenomenon of recent years, the fall in the mortality rate. That is to say, the development of effective chemotherapy in the early 1950s has not been the major influence on the incidence of the disease in the population, though it has vastly reduced the mortality among those suffering from it. *Per contra* the decline in incidence has had only a minor influence on mortality from the disease. The disease may therefore conveniently be considered either from the epidemiological point of view, with regard to its transmission in the population, or from the point of view of its pathological development in the individual patient. Both of these aspects are potentially important for an economic appraisal. The definition of a case is highly significant, and tends to be different according to whether it is considered from the epidemiological, the pathological or the economic point of view.

An infectious case infects a certain number of other people, and some of them become active cases, each subject to a certain degree of disability and to a certain risk of death. Some of these cases will become capable of passing the infection on to others. Various costs will be attached to this process, in terms of medical treatment, loss of income and amenity, etc. What is needed is an assessment of the values of the pathological and epidemiological parameters and of the various costs involved.

It would then be necessary to consider the effect of introducing MMR on all these. What effect would it have on the degree of disability, on the risk of death, on the costs attaching to all these and on the rate of infection if patients were diagnosed somewhat earlier by MMR? It cannot be claimed that we know the answers to these questions. Epidemiological research requires elaborate organisation and considerable outlay of money and skilled manpower. As a consequence, the available data tends to derive from widely different geographical, cultural and economic backgrounds, and it is not always clear how far the results obtained are comparable.

A Czechoslovakian investigation, which started in 1960, covered a population of about 100,000 and involved the biennial and triennial radiography of virtually the whole population.[10] During the first six years of the programme the prevalence of bacillary cases fell by half, from 150 to 73, but the number of newly discovered cases, though it fluctuated a great deal, fell only from 46 in the year before the study began to 44 six years later. The category regarded as of major epidemiological interest by the investigators, so far as the transmission of the disease is concerned, is that of persons excreting bacilli which can be found by direct miscroscopy.[11] The fall in the total of such cases from 80 to 34 was entirely accounted for by the fall in the number of chronic cases and relapses, the number of new cases remaining the same, at 21, in the last year as in the first. The conclusion was that, as a means of reducing the incidence, as opposed to the prevalence, of the disease, MMR is conspicuously ineffective even when used on a whole population.

Data on the average annual incidence of infection are available for the Netherlands.[12] These indicate that by the age of 14 about 80% of all infections to be expected up to the age of 50 have already occurred. This suggests that mass vaccination with BCG at the age of about 13, which costs about £100,000 a year in Britain, is likely to have a very much smaller effect in controlling the disease than if given earlier.

[10] K. Styblo, et al., 'Epidemiological and Clinical Study of Tuberculosis in the District of Kolin, Czechoslovakia', Bulletin of W.H.O., vol. 37, 1967, pp. 819–74.
[11] K. Styblo and I. Reil, 'Epidemiological Parameters of Tuberculosis', Scandinavian Journal of Respiratory Diseases, vol. 48, 1967, pp. 117–26.
[12] K. Styblo, J. Meijer and I. Sutherland, 'The Transmission of Tubercle Bacilli', Bulletin of the International Union against Tuberculosis, vol. 42, 1969, pp. 5–104.

The conclusion which emerges from these surveys, so far as incidence is concerned, seems to be that the economically justifiable course of action is to follow up contacts, possibly to maintain radiological surveillance of high-risk groups where co-operation can be obtained, and otherwise to allow the natural trends to continue. A satisfactory rate of self-referral is clearly implied by such a policy.

The findings of MMR tend to be rather unspecific. The exact significance of the index of specificity depends, of course, on how one defines a case, and this, in operational terms, depends on the further diagnostic tests applied to radiographic positives. From the epidemiological point of view emphasis tends to be placed on the direct microscopic investigation of sputum, but cultures and tuberculin tests may also be used diagnostically.

Although it is cases which are positive by direct microscopy which are important for transmission, other positive findings may be important in relation to the progression of the disease in the individual patient, and hence from the economic point of view also. Contrary to reasonable expectations, there exist data derived from a longitudinal study of cases without treatment, which enable some sort of view to be formed of the way in which the disease would have progressed among cases found by MMR if they had not been so found.[13]

It is hoped that this progression can be simulated by a probabilistic type of model, in which the probability that those in a given category in any period will find themselves in any particular category in the next period appears as an element in a transition matrix, the process continuing until determined by death or diagnosis.[14] To this matrix can then be applied a second, embodying the various 'costs' involved in being in a particular cell. This would simplify to a column vector if the current costs were assumed to depend only on the current state of the case, and not its previous states.

Unfortunately, the published data are not sufficiently complete to enable a fully satisfactory model to be easily developed.

A number of deaths from TB still occur, but mostly as the result of long-standing infections. In some cases notification (and hence

[13] Raj Narain et al., 'Problems of Defining a "Case" of Pulmonary Tuberculosis in Prevalence Surveys', Bulletin of W.H.O., vol. 39, 1968, No. 5, pp. 701–29.

[14] E. Fix and J. Neyman, 'A Simple Stochastic Model of Recovery, Relapse, Death and Loss of Patients', Human Biology, vol. 23, No. 3, September 1951, pp. 205–41.

presumably diagnosis) takes place *post mortem*, and there is some suggestion that a certain amount of over-reporting of deaths may occur, for various institutional reasons.

The general view among chest physicians appears to be that, so far as morbidity and mortality are concerned, the stage at which the disease is picked up is of very marginal significance. Apart from chronic and drug-resistant cases, rates of cure approach 100% provided adequate therapy is applied. Errors of treatment will no doubt continue to be made, but it does not appear likely that the incidence of errors or their consequences would be significantly different as a result of earlier diagnosis through MMR.

The degree of disability caused by TB is not usually very great nowadays, and is primarily determined by the size of the tubercular lesion. Most lesions found by MMR are insignificant in terms of actual disability, so that there may be some benefit here.

CONCLUSION

This study may be seen as making an attempt at the use of medical data to evaluate the complex of costs and benefits arising from a particular medical activity. Medical people obviously have a capacity to judge many issues intuitively which laymen have not; but if cost-effectiveness criteria are to be applied to health services, some formal analysis of the medical benefits as well as the costs seems to be inevitable. Whether economists are best suited to this task is perhaps open to question, but someone must surely try.

The further application of such analysis depends on the degree of success which can be achieved, but the field, even as far as public health programmes are concerned, is very wide. It is notable that, even in the case of tuberculosis, with its vast specialist literature, the present study could hardly have been contemplated as recently as five years ago. It would be interesting to know how far recent epidemiological investigations have been inspired by economic considerations.

COMMENT ON 'THE ECONOMICS OF MASS RADIOGRAPHY'

J. R. SHANNON
University of York

Mr Pole's paper is both stimulating and provocative. It successfully exposes and illustrates many of the issues, conceptual and practical, which bedevil economic analysis in the area which includes mass miniature radiography itself and screening programmes in general.

All I can do here is to bring out some points which I feel need particular emphasis, without being over-technical; matters which I believe will benefit from a continuing dialogue between economists and medical experts.

But first perhaps, and aside, Mr Pole begins his paper with a quotation from A. L. Cochrane and V. Springett which includes the phrase: '. . . One approach to the problem is the *purely economic* one' (my italics). The use of 'purely economic' is, I believe, subtly misleading. It implies to the layman a much narrower vision of the subject matter of economics than is necessarily the case. In a thorough appraisal of alternative resource-allocation possibilities the economist will wish to take into account *all* the differential effects which flow from the alternative possibilities; some of which effects are not generally seen by the layman as 'economic'. But in that they alter the satisfactions or dissatisfactions that people derive from their myriad activities (or even only their potential satisfactions), any such effects must be counted in somehow. This 'counting in' may of course be in the form of enumeration rather than evaluation.

Mr Pole says that pulmonary TB was chosen for a first exercise because it was a screenable disease for which the data—both medical and economic—appeared likely to be most abundant and reliable. Thus an attempt is made to see how far economic appraisal, addressed in particular to the question of when the screening programme should be terminated, can go in the most favourable circumstances.

My initial worry—and this is not to disparage the analysis in the

115

paper, but rather concerns the prospects for applying similar analysis elsewhere to elucidate 'higher level' allocation questions regarding, for example, how much to spend on TB prevention rather than cancer prevention—concerns the 'typicality' or otherwise of TB with respect to certain features which make for ease of programme appraisal in this sort of way. My impression is that TB is in fact rather an exceptional condition in some ways which I shall describe; and that even with these atypical features, the problems of appraisal, particularly in the evaluation of the benefits, remain enormous.

It is interesting to reflect that one of the quite unpredictable but unfortunate costs of the successful TB screening programmes in the past may well have been a premature and ill-considered leap, in the euphoria its success created, into other screening programmes of much more dubious value. In what ways may TB be exceptional among diseases and conditions for which screening programmes have been seriously advocated?

1. It is—or was—a relatively common disease, about which, one understands, the natural history is pretty thoroughly known.
2. It is a clear-cut condition which can at almost all stages be unambiguously distinguished from normality (unlike some other widespread conditions for which screening has been advocated, such as diabetes and anaemia).
3. Crucially—and as Mr Pole says, the controversy about other screening programmes relates mainly to the effectiveness of their early treatment—in the case of pulmonary TB there exist proven, acceptable treatments.

These characteristics that I have mentioned do not however apply simultaneously to almost any other disease or condition for which screening has been suggested. In the case of many of the cancers, for example, extraordinarily little is known about the natural histories of the conditions, and the effectiveness of their early treatment seems frequently to be the subject of hot dispute.

In the case of anaemia, Cochrane and Elwood have said: '. . . the situation is a bizarre one. Investigation into the value of screening for a well-known disease led to considerable doubt as to whether the disease exists.'[1] They conclude by saying that 'with our present know-

[1] Nuffield Provincial Hospitals Trusts, *Screening in Medical Care. Reviewing the Evidence*, London 1968, p. 93 (O.U.P.).

ledge, it is impossible to estimate gains as no evidence is available . . . until further research is completed no quantitative comparison is possible'. One hates to have to say, 'further research is needed'; but it is my firm belief at present, and one would suspect Mr Pole's too, that the biggest obstacle at the moment to useful economic analysis of diseases and their prevention, is the sheer lack of medical know-ledge about diseases' natural histories and the effects of treatments on disablement, debility and death. Until a lot more *is* known, one doubts that economists will be able to do much intellectually satisfy-ing *applied* work. In the particular case of the economic appraisal of screening for TB, the usefulness of the exercise must be diminished to some extent by the fact that there exist few other programmes which are evaluable with which it can be compared.

A central problem, to which frequent allusion has been made at this conference, is that only some of the benefits (and indeed costs) can be measured with any sort of degree of precision. The danger of course is that the intangibles (e.g. the benefits of less pain, physical and psychic, both to the individual and the family) may well in truth overwhelm the measurable benefits yet be ignored because they are not put down in hard figures. It is the problem of what one economist has likened to that of appraising the quality of horse and rabbit stew. The horse, here being the amalgam of external effects, the social, emotional and psychological impacts, swamps rabbit, here those few consequences numerically measurable. If the effect of the horse in the stew swamps that of the rabbit, why waste much valuable time and effort in attempting meticulously to evaluate the rabbit?

One answer to this, and a good answer, is that if someone does pay for the stew (or the hospital or the old peoples' home), and if one can find out the value of the rabbit component, the purchaser can be told that he must value the 'intangible' horse element by *at least* the difference between the total price and his valuation of the rabbit. Such information, given to the purchaser can surely only help him in his future decisions.

Thus, to the critic of the economist who attempts to evaluate the returns to investment in, say, mental hospitals, the economist can point out that what he *can* attempt usefully to do is to inform the decision-maker how much he is implicitly evaluating humanitarian motives, charity, etc. The decision-maker may well find in the light of such information that, taking into consideration other public expenditure programmes both within the health sector and outside it, he is being inconsistent in the pursuit of his objectives. Inconsistencies, if these relate to arguments in the decision-maker's objective function, must almost certainly mean inefficiencies exist, even if one doesn't know precisely what global efficiency entails. Very often, one might be able to specify at least the *direction* of increased efficiency.

A final comment on the costing side. Sometimes workers in this field, and one finds particularly non-economists, tend to think that the costing side is simply a matter of adding up the published figures (salaries, drug expenditures, etc.). But in a service characterised by its non-market nature, our suspicion must be that the prices of inputs that we observe, do not in general reflect the opportunity costs of employing these factors. Nor indeed are relative prices likely to reflect relative opportunity costs. It may be that the shadow prices that we should employ are extremely difficult to calculate; and of course, observed prices are often used even by those who accept the naïvete of doing so. But it should be stressed that the general tendency to think 'costs easy, benefits difficult', is a dangerous and misleading one.

In conclusion: one feels that the TB case does seem in several ways to be atypical, and that even with its favourable features, the problems of cost and benefit evaluation seem enormous. However if we are prepared to operate on the rough principle that if anything we overestimate costs and underestimate benefits, useful economic appraisal, in the manner which Mr Pole suggests, does seem possible.

SOME STUDIES OF THE CONSEQUENCES OF REALLOCATION AND RELOCATION OF FUNCTION WITHIN THE COMMUNITY HEALTH SERVICES

J. M. BEVAN

Faculty of Social Sciences, University of Kent

INTRODUCTION

The work of the health services is undertaken from many centres in an area. Some are large with elaborate equipment and their staff are mostly occupied with activities within the centres. Others are small with little by way of specialised facilities and partly serve as bases for fairly mobile staff who do much of their work in ordinary homes.

The title of this paper refers to the reallocation and relocation of functions within the health service. Who should do what, where and when?

There is clearly a whole range of problems concerned with the roles respectively of the hospital and the community health services, and decisions concerning these will to a large extent determine the type of premises and equipment provided for the community health services. The advent of more sophisticated plant and especially automation has led to a centralisation of hospital facilities in a relatively small number of large units. As the hospital service has, however, returned to these central bastions it would seem to have taken with it most if not all of the responsibilities acquired when it was more widely dispersed. Indeed, the possibility of more accurate diagnosis and more effective treatment associated with the development of medical science and technology, has continued to give impetus to the centralisation of medical activity at the hospital.

Because of the costly nature of modern hospital treatment and its geographical inconvenience for patients, there is a counter trend toward modifying the community health services in such a way as to reduce to a minimum the element in the hospital load that does not specifically require hospital facilities—especially since it is likely that even the demand for hospital care modified in this way will be as great as, if not more than, that which can be supplied.

The possibility that the community health services may have to take over more of the work currently carried on within hospitals is an additional stimulus for seeing whether work can be distributed more appropriately within these services. Doctors take a long time to train and are expensive to run. To what extent are their skills fully used in general practice? How much of the work can be properly delegated to other personnel? What are the consequences of such delegation? The same questions can be asked about the work of para-medical and other personnel in the community health services.

The question 'where?' arises in two connections: (i) what sort of premises should the community health service personnel work from and (ii) how mobile should such personnel be in the sense of working away from the base premises?

SOME GENERAL REMARKS ON STUDIES OF INNOVATION

(The word 'innovation' is used to denote the new scheme which is being evaluated.)

Some existing and perhaps new personnel will be actively involved in the innovation. The work they do may change in nature and quantity, both directly due to the innovation and indirectly due to its external repercussions.[1] Thus, for example, if it becomes easier by virtue of the innovation to obtain a service, more people may in time take the trouble to seek it. Parts of the health service outside that in which the innovation has taken place may also be affected by the change.

If patients or other consumers are directly involved how are they informed, if at all, of the innovation? How does it affect their feeling about the service and their relationships with the personnel involved? No less important is what happens to the personnel directly involved in the area of innovation. How do their relationships with one another change and how do individual members of the group see their jobs and those of their colleagues in the light of the change?

[1] The nature of the work of new staff brought in because of the innovation may be even less predictable.

The character of the changes induced by the innovation may vary with the quantity and type of work falling upon the part of the service in which it is made.[2]

Changes may slowly but steadily manifest themselves or there may be a gestation period followed by a sudden change (depending perhaps on the nature of the learning process). Or, yet again, some external or catalytic trigger mechanism may bring into being changes potentially to be found in a situation (e.g. a change in the constraints upon the activities of certain personnel).[3]

It is clear that even if an innovation is made at one point in the system it can cause reverberations over other parts. If, moreover, changes are going on all over the place, both those that are intended and those that just happen, these may interact in quite complicated ways so that it is difficult to unravel the tangle of cause-effect relationships.

The empirical study of the effects of trying out some innovation is thus full of pitfalls; yet to fail to make some such study is to rely on subjective views of the effects in question, which may be still less reliable. A controlled experiment even in the limited sense of the clinical or agricultural trial, is seldom possible. Cross-sectional studies in which one studies the situation at a given point of time over a wide range of units (in this context including some which have the relevant innovation and some that have not), clearly run into difficulties because of the wide variation between individual sites[4] within the health services which may well swamp all but the most extreme differences arising from having or not having the studied innovation.

Moreover, the fact that the consequences of an innovation may often take some time to manifest themselves fully is a further disadvantage of confining an enquiry to a given point in time. One can get information from different respondents about innovations that have been in operation for various periods of time, but not about the same unit over a period of time (except by asking the respondent to recall what happened). None the less, cross-sectional studies may usefully complement other approaches to provide information

---

[2] See: Royal College of General Practitioners, *The Practice Nurse*, Reports from General Practice, No. 10, London 1968.
[3] Ibid.
[4] I.e. of investigation.

economically on attitudes of people involved in the innovations over a wide range of situations, and subjective assessments of what happened. Very little hard data can, however, be acquired using this method in this context.

Longitudinal studies, in which some sites making the innovation and some not are studied over a period of time, do go some way toward answering the problem associated with the time which some phenomena take to reveal themselves; but again the other differences between the sites in the study may obscure the effects of innovation. Before-and-after studies, in which a number of sites are studied before the innovation is made and again afterward, do have the advantage that one can study the consequences of innovation *within* a site, so screening out between site variation. It may sometimes be sensible not to rely only on before-and-after studies in sites making an innovation, otherwise one may fail to discern general trends and so confuse what is happening because of the innovation with what is happening anyway. By studying the sites concerned for a sufficient time before and after the innovation, not necessarily with uniform intensity, one may be able to get some insight into trends other than those directly concerned with the innovation.

The trouble associated with the longitudinal and, in particular, before-and-after studies is the sheer cost in terms of time and analysis. If it is agreed that the consequences of an innovation may be complex and hard to extricate from the general developments in a situation, it follows that the nature of the data to be collected must be appropriately sophisticated. Since this inevitably involves the people working at the site of the innovation in a lot of extra labour, or they have to be closely observed, this in itself limits the opportunity to conduct such enquiries. Participants in the studies are either enthusiasts or at least are willing to be persuaded to take on the extra work. There is no guarantee that such people are typical of their colleagues in general. Again, being investigated and perhaps thinking about what is happening as a result of the innovation can affect the nature of one's work. On grounds other than research this has been suggested as a good reason for undertaking such studies.

These gloomy observations emphasise the need for extreme care in the conduct of studies of innovation in the organisational sphere and in their interpretation. Consistency is perhaps what one is looking for in one's results: consistency between results arising from different sites and research methods and between the results of different research organisations; consistency if one has a plausible model with the predictions it offers; consistency more generally with what common sense suggests. Apparently freak results are always a bit disquieting and can force one to call into question the methods used in the study. Then there is internal consistency in the overall body of findings emerging from the study. This is not to say that inconsistency between results from different sites is a ground for abandoning the study. To know why the inconsistency arises is, however, important. Perhaps people are adopting different conventions in keeping records or questions are understood in different ways in different places. Perhaps however there are local conditions which interact with the innovation to give rise to the inconsistency. So far, in talking about between-site variation one has been talking about this as a kind of nuisance. However, often one of the main aims of a study is to examine the effects of variations in conditions—e.g. size and complexity of local organisation, environment—on the operation of the innovation. Hence the need for the study to cover a range of sites representative of those in which it is hoped to institute the innovation on a regular basis. The annoying variation is that which arises between sites which are apparently similar with respect to the features deemed to be important.

A REVIEW OF SOME STUDIES OF INNOVATION

An Innovation with Few Side Effects[5]
Appointment systems in GPs' surgeries seem to be fairly common these days but in the early 1960s only about 10% of doctors had been converted to their use, though there seemed to be quite a lot of professional interest in the idea. By that time several papers had been written by GPs on their appointment system mostly favourable. Quite a lot of work, theoretical and empirical, had been devoted to the study of hospital appointment systems,[6] which in turn arose out of

[5] J. M. Bevan and G. J. Draper, *Appointment Systems in General Practice*, The Nuffield Provincial Hospitals Trust, London 1967 (O.U.P.).
[6] E.g. N. T. J. Bailey, 'A Study of Queues and Appointment Systems in Hospitals Out-Patient Departments, with Special Reference to Waiting Times', *Journal of the Royal Statistical Society*, Series B, vol. 14, 1952, p. 185.

studies in the branch of probabilistic mathematics known as queueing theory.[7]

Because of this activity the sort of thing that one might expect to happen when an appointment system was introduced had been widely discussed. What seemed to be needed was a conclusive answer to the question from an individual doctor, or for that matter, patient: 'if an appointment system were introduced in my surgery, would it really stand a good chance of doing all the nice things it is supposed to do?'.

In particular, on a broadly mechanical level:

1. What would happen to the number of patients in the waiting-room during surgery hours?
2. To what extent would patients' waiting time be reduced?
3. How far would it be possible to control the times and days when patients attended the surgery?
4. How punctual would patients be when attending by appointment?
5. How many would use the appointment system (this was at a time when quite a lot of stress was laid on the fact that the patient did not have to make an appointment though he would be encouraged to do so)?
6. How much would the appointment system cost to run?
7. What were the staffing implications?

A number of questions arose on some of the less-direct possible consequences of such an innovation. For example:

8. What would be the effect of the appointment system on the doctor's overall workload?
9. How would the time discipline implicit in the appointment system affect the doctor's way of working in the surgery—the content of his work, average consulting time, etc.?
10. Would the use of a receptionist to organise appointments and so potentially to control access to the doctor, put a barrier between the doctor and the patients (and indeed create a new sort of para-medical job)?

It would also be of interest to know what the various people—patients, receptionists and doctors—who were involved in appointment systems thought of them. Equally important, especially if it

[7] D. R. Cox and W. L. Smith, *Queues*, London 1961 (Methuen).

should prove that an appointment system was a generally desirable innovation, was what those who did not have such a system knew and thought about the idea. (Questioning people, especially patients, about something outside their direct experience is clearly a difficulty in this respect.) Information required for the study was collected from:

(a) a small series of before-and-after studies;
(b) a survey among practices using appointment systems;
(c) a survey among doctors not using appointment systems; and
(d) two surveys, one postal and the other by interview, among the general public.

The object of the before-and-after studies was to provide the hard data necessary to answer questions about, for example, the punctuality of patients, changes in numbers in the waiting-room, waiting times of patients, proportion of patients attending by appointment, changes in the nature and magnitude of load including the ratio of home visits to surgery attendances.

About a dozen practices were involved in this part of the study. The amount of variety one can incorporate within so small a number is limited, but an attempt was made to include practices of various sizes, in various settings, urban and rural, north and south. Whilst the practices were self-selected insofar that they were a subset of those intending to start appointment systems, an attempt was made to recruit practices which were not especially enthusiastic about research or record keeping.

Records of various kinds were kept, usually for a month before the appointment system, and for two further periods of a month (separated by a few months) afterward; the most intensive and harrowing of the records was kept for only one week in each of these months. It might be argued that these last were very small intervals of time upon which to base any conclusions, and perhaps not worth bothering about at all. Consistent and plausible results were, however, obtained. Also, since the intensive record-keeping weeks were carried out at different times of the year, more or less haphazardly for different practices, no consistent bias due to calendar effect might be expected. One could also compare the intensive weeks with the other weeks in which records were kept to some extent, to see how typical they were.

Granted the limitations of this approach, one was able to show certain consistent results. Average waiting times were reduced to about half their pre-appointment system values. Quite high proportions of the patients attended by appointment and, though not all were perfect time-keepers, the great majority arrived not later than five minutes after their appointment times. The numbers in the waiting-room declined, the decline being predictably the most marked in practices where most patients came by appointment. Equally interesting were the apparent non-changes; workloads seemed in general little changed and there seemed insufficient evidence to suggest a change generally in the ratio of home visits to surgery attendances.

By recourse to the survey among doctors using appointment systems one was, at least at a subjective level, able to check some of the hard data-based findings of the before-and-after studies, and in addition to find out: something more generally about the costs of operating systems; certain details relating to the method of introduction and type of appointment system used; and impressions on some of the less easily measurable possible effects of an appointment system. Thus, for example, this survey confirmed the finding that the overall workload and, in particular, home visit levels were little changed for the majority, though over a quarter did report a decline in the number of home visits requested by patients. Most respondents, especially those with full appointment systems, were well satisfied with their systems, believing them to achieve the direct 'scheduling' objects for which they were introduced. The majority view was that such indirect or side effects (e.g. effects on doctor-patient relationship, strain on doctors, etc.) as were evident were beneficial to practice life. The overall impression received was that an appointment system was a useful scheduling mechanism which made life easier for most of those involved in the work of the practice (patient and doctor) with no profound side effects on the relationship and nature and quality of work. Most thought that appointment systems were easy to institute regardless of the social background of patients.

The other survey among doctors probed the reasons which decided doctors against introducing appointment systems. A by-product associated with this study was the unexpected discovery that about 10% of practices starting appointment systems abandoned them often with great relief afterward. It then became important to find out why appointment systems sometimes did not succeed—was it due to local circumstances, individual tastes or what? An informal study was mounted into this as a result.

Another fact that emerged was that the existing methods of re-imbursement of GPs' expenses did have some deterrent effect as far as starting appointment systems was concerned among small practices, especially the single-handed. These last were also at a disadvantage in the sense that, although receptionist cover was needed, at least during surgery hours, the need was not for a fully occupied recep-tionist per doctor but rather for the presence of somebody. Econom-ies of scale relating to indivisibility of resources were particularly in evidence in this sphere.

In the case of patient surveys, particular importance was attached to the consistency of results—initially within each of the surveys and between the two surveys, conducted as they were in radically different ways. Both surveys revealed that substantially more people were in favour of appointment systems at their doctor's surgery when their doctor actually ran one than was the case for those whose doctor did not. Now this is only partly comforting because there is a tendency for people to support the *status quo*. Confidence in at least the qualitative validity of this sort of statement was increased by the consideration of several further pieces of evidence:

1. Among those whose doctor did *not* run an appointment system but who had previously attended a doctor who did, the propor-tion of those in favour of appointment systems was almost exactly the same as in the case of those whose doctor currently used an appointment system.
2. Support of the appointment system of their doctor was not un-critical and tended to sharply diminish for those who still had as a rule to wait a long time, by which they meant more than about fifteen minutes, after the appointment time.
3. Several findings including (2) were in accord with those of another independent worker.[8]

The study indicated that the 'higher' the respondent's class the more likely he was to be in favour of an appointment system, but the

[8] A. Cartwright, *Patients and their Doctors*, London 1967 (Routledge and Kegan Paul).

differences were not marked between classes except between the lowest income group and the rest. The aged also seemed somewhat less in favour of appointment systems than did younger people. Both the aged and those in the lowest income group (there is of course a good deal of overlap) were, however, much more likely to be in favour of appointment systems when their doctor ran one than when their doctor did not.

The problem of what to measure was perhaps not too critical in this study. The proportion of new or patient-initiated attendances by appointment as a measure of patient support of the system, was important. The precise definition of punctuality (arrival not later than five minutes after appointment time) also clarified the picture. A useful definition of 'numbers' in the waiting-room was also required.

The study of appointment systems in a sense was relatively straightforward. It appeared in most cases that the effect of the appointment system was limited to cutting down waiting times and the numbers in the waiting-room and regulating the flow of patients through the day and week. It did not appear to have wider ranging effects on the structure of the GP's work etc. That is not to say that it might not ultimately have had some such effect; systems are seldom static. The receptionist is no longer in any way an unusual phenomenon in even the smallest practice and the advent of the medical secretary or nurse-receptionist emphasises the possibility in an appointment system practice, of the receptionist's taking on a screening function. Again the effect of an appointment system depends on the objective one has in introducing it. If it is solely to regulate the flow of patients in the surgery it may well have no other effect. If, however, it is introduced specifically with a view to, say, reducing the proportion of consultations at home, then the manner in which it is operated may well produce the desired effect—compare the biased and unbiased question in a questionnaire.

A Study of Delegation

A project carried out by members of the North East Faculty of the Royal College of General Practitioners, in one sense came about as near to an experiment as possible in this sort of enquiry in that four practices in North East England were persuaded to take on practice nurses (to be financed for the duration of the enquiry by the then

Ministry of Health). The practices were all urban but of various sizes ranging from a partnership of five to a single-handed practice strictly one and one-third doctors). All but one used an appointment system. At the time when appointment systems were still rare one wondered whether this was unfortunate, though it could be argued that since the trend has been toward appointment systems the study is the more valid for being ahead of its time in this respect. Against this comforting thought is the possibility that we were dealing with a band of innovating doctors, not typical therefore of their colleagues. In the event it appeared from the limited evidence available that the practice without an appointment system did not produce results that were essentially different from those of the other three.

The rationale for concentrating the whole study in the North East, apart from convenience, was that certain difficulties were thought to be present in this situation, so that if the innovation worked there it would work anywhere. One aspect of the study was to determine whether it was possible to recruit otherwise unemploy-able[9] nurses and practice nurses and these were thought to be in relatively short supply in the North East—in the end though, four nurses of high quality were recruited without too much difficulty. List sizes were fairly large in this area and the premises from which at least two of the practices under study were working were rather limited.

The field-work of the study consisted of a recording period of a month before the nurses started work, followed by two further periods several months and a year later respectively (to allow time for nurses to settle into their jobs). As it happened, the before period took place rather hurriedly before full agreement had been obtained on classification definitions by the participants. For one practice the period of record keeping coincided with something of a 'flu' outbreak.

There is a lot to be said for making sure that the before period is as fully and representatively studied as possible, since one cannot go back later.

Basically, the doctors timed their consultations in the home and surgery and also other aspects of their work—travel and administration—and recorded certain details of each consultation: whether new, acute return, chronic return or a procedure (a confusing

[9] E.g. due to family commitments.

E

category), diagnosis[10] and whether nurses could have done the item of work. The nurse recorded essentially the same information in respect of her consultations. The nurse was not permitted to see new cases but otherwise attended patients in the surgery and at home, nearly always unaccompanied by the doctor. The type of work she was to do was carefully laid down, as was the regime for briefing by and reporting to the doctor so that the management of cases remained securely in the latter's hands. It was also agreed that the nurses should only do work which the doctors would have had to do in their absence and not attempt to do new things, e.g. additional screening.

There was a good deal of scepticism on the part of the doctors participating at first about whether a nurse could do much of anything the doctor currently did, and this was reflected in the small proportion of consultations (in terms of time and numbers) which they recorded as appropriate for the nurse to undertake. This view changed a good deal once the nurses were installed and by the recording session a year later the nurses were working for seven to ten hours per week per doctor. The doctors recorded that hardly any of their remaining work was of a sort appropriate for the nurse to undertake.

The original idea was that the nurse would 'save' the doctor's time. But was this a meaningful concept? The doctors spent about the same time at their work in normal circumstances after the nurse had joined the practice as before. This seems to be in accord with Parkinson's Law.[11] But how did the doctors spend their time? They saw rather fewer patients but spent more time on average per consultation. It was intended that the nurse should particularly concentrate on certain chronic and acute return consultations and deal with all 'consultations' which were categorised as procedures, by which was meant 'that something was done but no consultation in the real sense of the word took place'. The nurse did appear to make some inroads into the practice workload in these three categories, though by no means all the procedure-type work disappeared from the doctors' load (even though the residue was not categorized as appropriate for the nurse—confusion of definition here?). This conclusion was based on:

[10] Categorised according to the Royal College of General Practitioners' eighteen major diseases classification.

[11] See Hodgkin and Gillie in *The Practice Nurse, loc. cit.*

(a) an apparent decline in the number of such consultations made by the doctor when the nurse was working in the practice, compared with the pre-nurse situation, and

(b) the content of the nurses' workload.

Because the nurses undertook some of the practice visiting, a by-product of their presence was a reduction in the driving time of the doctors. Indeed this seemed to be the area of activity in which the nurse really saved most doctor-time. The reverse applied to administration time, which increased quite definitely with the advent of the nurse due to a need for briefing sessions etc. (In one practice the increase in administrative time totally overwhelmed any saving of the doctors' time in other respects!)

All this raised the question of whether it was inappropriate to think of all time saved as of equal value. If the nurses could save the doctor time by reducing his driving time, this is fairly clearly a gain because the doctor has been relieved of work which in no way utilises his special skills (nor the nurse's for that matter). Equally, if the increase in administrative time is concerned with wider discussion of cases by doctors and nurses, this may well make for better medicine.

We do not know of course how the extra administrative time arose for we had not attempted any subdivision of administrative time. It did appear though that the practice whose administrative time had increased most markedly ascribed this increase to a daily case conference which did have a partly educative role. To some extent, 'administrative' time can be made to vary according to the other more strictly medical demands made on the practice. It may even be a form of relaxation to some people.

Again, does an increase in average consulting time imply rising standards of care? Hodgkin[12] has pointed out that by relieving the pressure on the doctor the nurse was providing a useful service—the actual benefit being greatest when a practice was working at capacity. The higher the case load the more 'frills' (i.e. non-basic or non-urgent elements) the doctor had to abandon. The presence of a nurse to whom he could delegate work meant that not so much had to be abandoned.

This brings us back to the problem of what one should be measuring in attempting to assess the effect of a nurse on a practice's work.

[12] In *The Practice Nurse* Study, *loc. cit.*

To count the number of consultations in various categories which the nurse undertakes seems simple and relevant. It establishes at least a lower limit for the nurse's capacity to undertake items of work. To look at the absolute number of doctors' consultations before and after the coming of the nurse in the corresponding categories, helps to put the data on the nurse's workload into perspective and enables one to check some assumed constants of the study. Measuring the time spent by the doctors and nurses respectively on various parts of their work enables one:

(a) to see how the doctor redistributes his time;
(b) to determine the number of nurse-hours required by practices of various sizes per week;
(c) to compare the rates of working of doctor and nurse for activities in similar categories (in general the nurse's average consulting time was rather larger than the doctor's—though this may have been due to the nurse's seeing relatively few patients per week—since in the one practice where her load was of the same magnitude as the doctor's this was not so);
(d) to provide an upper bound to the quantity of time saved for the doctors by the nurse (this cannot exceed, unless one postulates positive interactive effects, the total time worked by the nurse); and
(e) to see the relative importance of different items when it comes to easing the workload, e.g. a home visit saved means the saving of time spent consulting and some travelling time.

But a knowledge of the numbers of consultations and the time taken to carry out various times of work, only enables one to guess at the more general effects on the practice of the doctor's delegating part of his workload. The doctors participating in the study were very conscious of the reduction of fatigue and a feeling of being less under pressure following the introduction of the nurse into the practices. Again, what was the effect of the innovation, if any, on the actual health of the practice population involved? It is not easy to discern a change in the quality of medical care, even if one could easily measure or conceptualise it, due to an innovation, without a fairly long and full period of record keeping. In some ways it is an easier task to find out whether patients think they are being better or worse cared for as a result of an innovation. (Nothing formal was done in this respect—largely because of the heavy outlay of time required and because there were no research staff working full time at all on this project.)

One practice among those studied, subsequently carried out some work study on their methods of operation and made a number of changes. Also, the nurse was used for primary visiting in certain well-defined cases (thus one constraint was removed). The combined impact of the nurses' contribution and the organisation changes, appeared much greater than those observed as due to the presence of the nurse only. It is difficult to be more precise when the result is based on one practice during a voluntary extra recording session, but the findings seem reasonable and emphasise the point that an innovation may not realise its full value unless the system into which it is introduced is optimised or re-optimised.

Postscript. One was interested to see whether some very simple models could be fitted to the data of the study. In connection with driving time it was clear that, other things being equal, the greater the number of visits, the lower the average distance (and so driving time) between them. There appeared to be some theoretical grounds for trying a relationship[13] of the form $T_d = a + bn^{\frac{1}{2}}$ where T_d was total driving time and n the number of calls in the week. This fitted quite well for the very limited data available for the two practices, in which it was tried. A somewhat similar exercise attempting to relate time spent consulting (T_c) to the number of consultations per week (n) using $T_c = a + b/n$ was less successful. Hopeful as these relationships looked as far as estimating with appropriate confidence intervals the time saved due to a nurse's presence, assuming that she took various loads of work (number of consultations), the situation is complicated by the fact that while it is possible to provide pessimistic and very wide limits, more realistic limits need to be approached via a study of the underlying structure giving rise to the model (this is currently being investigated).

A Study on Relocation

GPs spend a lot of time travelling in the course of visiting patients (often about 7–10 hours per week, excluding the actual time of the

[13] See, e.g., J. Beardwood, J. H. Halton and J. M. Hammersley, 'The Shortest Path through many Points', *Proceedings Cambridge Philosophical Society*, vol. 55, 1959, p. 299.

consultation). This caused a number of people to examine the scope for reducing what is essentially wasted doctor-hours of time spent in this way. One of the practices in the Practice Nurse Study started zoning its visiting during the study period, a fact which complicated the analysis of the effects of the nurse but did suggest that quite considerable savings of time could be effected in this way.[14] Floyd[15] and colleagues operate a practice minibus service in an urban practice and patients who telephone before 10 a.m. for a home visit are offered the alternative of a consultation in the surgery with travel both ways by the minibus. A high proportion accept this (currently about half). Quite apart from any saving of doctors' time arising from this, Floyd reported that many patients who had found it difficult to get out at all prior to the minibus service seemed much the better for the occasional trip to the surgery.

A group of doctors practising from a small country town served by a very limited bus service observed that they were visiting many people in their homes because they had no means of getting to the surgery. A study was therefore carried out for two periods each of a month, in which certain details were obtained for all persons attended by the doctors at home or in the surgeries, main or branch. Similar details were collected for the nurse who worked in the main surgery. Information was collected on the nature of the consultation, address code,[16] age, sex and marital status of the patients, transport facilities available to them and possible items which might tie them to the house; there was also one item on the need for patients to attend surgery anyway because of their need for the specialised facilities available there (the main surgery was in a fairly sophisticated building with many facilities available). Analysis of the study is still not complete but it is clear that the doctors differed a good deal in the proportion of home visits designated as not necessary on medical grounds, i.e. the people who might be brought to the surgery if transport were available (proportions ranged from 4 to 54%). They

[14] The doctors did between them an average 11 hours per week less driving (20 as compared with 31) after zoning and the nurse were introduced but the nurse only averaged 1½ hours travelling time per week—total patients seen had however declined by a sixth only.

[15] C. B. Floyd, 'Car Service in General Practice: A Two-Year Survey', *British Medical Journal*, vol. 2, 1968, pp. 614–17. Originally a car, not a minibus, was used.

[16] The practice area was divided into twenty-six 'sites' roughly corresponding to a village or a ward of town.

were agreed however that the 'over 60s' were the most likely to be in this situation and, in fact, 44% of the persons visited were in this age group. Predictably, the proportion of those visited who lived out of town who could have attended surgery if transport had been available was slightly greater than the corresponding proportion for those who lived in town.

An attempt is being made in this study to assess the potential for time saving by laying on a transport service and so removing from the visiting rounds the patients visited on the grounds of lack of transport only. The method employed is first to build up from the data a 'table' of average times taken to travel between and within sites in the doctor's area with their standard errors. One will then be able to examine average times taken to travel along the paths corresponding to doctors' rounds in a given period and to compare these with the average times for the paths obtained by removing unnecessary visits and re-optimising. Optimal paths can be calculated from a knowledge of times taken to traverse the individual links. The average time saved here with attendant standard error is strictly that applicable if the doctors had the same visiting patterns, trimmed of unnecessary visiting, as those in the study. Clearly if they were to reorganise their rounds so as to be of the same size or larger than the 'untrimmed' rounds, they might save additional time as they might if zoning were adopted.

Analysis of the sort described might be carried out in the course of examining other similar problems, e.g. in the course of determining the benefit and costs of consultants coming to health centres and consulting there as opposed to patients staying in hospital. (Also compare this sort of analysis with PERT.)

When translating time saved into costs saved, once again one is faced with the problem of what is done with the spare time. There is a sense in which the cutting out of unnecessary work done by the doctor, like driving, could yield direct savings in the long run in that estimates of the numbers of doctors needed overall could be revised in the light of projected saving of time. The effect of cutting down doctors' travelling time and so opening the possibility of reducing the number of doctors needed for a given population,[17] has implications for the use of practice premises in that the bringing of more patients to the surgery means that the doctors will be consulting

[17] To maintain the same standard of care.

longer in the surgery and so making fuller use of the plant and at the same time there would be less of them.[18] It is arguable that the number of doctors in a health centre (rather than the number of patients for which they are responsible) is one of the most important considerations in fixing the size of the centre.

The question of delegating some of the doctor's non-specialised tasks to non-specialised people brings out the paradox that, while the doctor can usually do a large number of things (not just medical) very well, he ought to be the least flexible person in the community health team. This is because people with his skills are in short supply and cost a lot (the two are not necessarily the same). Conversely, staff with the minimum of specialised skills ought to be encouraged to maintain the maximum flexibility acceptable to all concerned in the work they do.

Monitoring a Move
The studies so far discussed have each been concerned with one specific innovation. The final study to be described is concerned with a change less well-defined. What happens when several family doctors and other workers move from their traditional-type premises into a purpose-built medical centre? This was the situation examined in a small industrial town in the North East involving six principals from three practices who were moving into a centre incorporated in the new shopping centre of the town. What does this change actually consist of? There has been a change of location from side streets to town centre; from several sites to one. (The distances involved were all about one quarter of a mile.) Then there is the fact that doctors used to practising in relative isolation are now brought into a group and see more of one another, if only at coffee in the common room. There is usually likely to be more than one of them about the centre at the time. The premises are generally more pleasant and better equipped and staffed.

What results might all this have? A change of location especially into the middle of the shopping centre might alter the nature and magnitude of the load and its spread during the day. Will more or less people come to the surgery now? Will more people seek home

[18] The waiting-area and appointment system may need some adaptation to accommodate the arrival of minibus loads of people, and the queues for it on its departure.

visits? Does the relatively complex establishment put off the elderly and the not too bright, whereas a surgery in a terraced house down the road does not? Again, the fact that the doctors are associated in a *de facto* group might mean that they have an effect on each other's way of practising. There might be a tendency toward homogeneity in a number of respects. Perhaps being in a group is reassuring. It is easier to get a second opinion and this might lead to doctors becoming more adventurous in their decisions. It is likely that as a group it is much easier to arrange rota systems for off-duty periods and so on. The concentration of doctors in a purpose-built centre will make them more of a force to be reckoned with when it comes to dealing with other parts of the health service, e.g. pathology laboratories may be prepared to lay on special transport services for a centre.

With so many possible effects, some of which could have arisen for several reasons associated with the move to the group practice, it is going to be difficult to unravel the cause-effect relationships. However, it seemed worthwhile making an attempt to see what happened in some respects. The method of attack was to adopt several methods of data collection, some formal, some highly informal. Data were collected about each consultation for a few weeks before the move into the new centre and for periods afterward. These data were concerned with the type of consultation and what action was taken during the course of it, a special interest being in the work referred to other parts of the health service. Details were also collected concerning the home location of patients and possible travelling problems. It has been arranged to obtain certain information on prescribing and also data from the local hospital unit on numbers of requests for X-rays and pathology. Doctors were questioned informally about what they thought would happen soon after they moved into the centre and a postal survey among patients was conducted. Certain simple counts of patients seen were available for longer periods before and after the move into the medical centre. It is hoped, when the centre has been functioning for a rather longer period, to question doctors and patients again. The analysis of the existing data is incomplete but some interim results are available which will serve to illustrate the sort of information obtainable from the study.

The overall workload in terms of the total number of patients seen by the doctors per week at home and in the surgery seemed virtually constant for all recording sessions. The proportion of patients who were seen at home in mid-summer 1969 was somewhat lower than that in mid-summer 1968. (This change, 17.1% as compared with 19.7%, was consistent for all but one doctor. It was not in evidence in the shorter recording session in early summer 1969.) The proportion of new consultations increased both at home and in the surgery. It will be interesting to see whether the suggestion in the data that the proportion of surgery new attendances had increased relatively quickly and then stabilised while the corresponding figures for home visits increased in a slower but steadier fashion, is borne out by later data from the centre (data for one practice on surgery attendances extending for six months before the centre opened and the same six months a year later did confirm this impression). For individual doctors the proportion of new surgery attendances ranged from 44 to 83% in mid-summer 1968 and from 61 to 79% in mid-summer 1969. Thus the increased proportion of new attendances can be explained by a tendency for the doctors to become more homogeneous in their practice rather than because of an overall move upward. This move toward homogeneity is probably a result of discussion by the doctors on their differing new/return consultation ratios—there was considerable interest in the subject.

Another aspect of the workload's falling upon the centre and local health services generally, was that arising out of consultations. Overall the proportion of consultations involving the taking of specimens increased from 2·8 to 4·4%, but in fact the increase was solely due to three doctors belonging to one practice; the figures for the others were effectively unchanged. A daily collection by the laboratory of pathology specimens was introduced following the opening of the medical centre. This could have been a possible stimulus for change. It would appear that some doctors were affected and some were not. Indeed the practice of the doctors in taking specimens became more heterogeneous.

If anything, the proportion of consultations involving X-rays declined following the move to the centre. It is not clear how far this can be ascribed, if at all, to the departure of the radiographer at the local chest clinic which was followed by a space before a new appointment was made during which the local X-ray unit's service was seriously curtailed.

In the medical centre 67% of patients at the surgery were seen at surgeries starting before 4 p.m., as compared with 52% in the recording session before the centre opened. This change is explained almost entirely by the increase in the proportion attending afternoon surgeries (this trend was something which the doctors at the centre wished to encourage).

The proportion of elderly patients (who might regard the centre least favourably) among those attending the surgery was 8·5% in the pre-centre recording period and 7·8% when the centre had opened. There was also some suggestion that a higher proportion of doctors' chronic return consultations were taking place at home. Some re-organisation of the district nurses' roles took place following the opening of the centre, which might have affected these figures. It is hoped that further analysis and enquiry may throw some light on this matter.

The proportion of patients attending the surgery by bus increased from 26·7% in the pre-centre days to 32·2% during the recording sessions when the centre was open, while there was a greater than corresponding decline in the proportion walking. This was a consistent finding for five of the six principals participating in the study. Travelling distances probably had not changed greatly for most patients though they were more likely to encounter a bus route leading toward the centre than toward the old surgery premises.

Among the questions asked in the 1968 survey of people on the lists of the doctors moving into the centre, were a couple designed to investigate how strongly people wanted to see their own doctor. It appeared that women were much more strongly attached to their doctor than men and that older people of both sexes were both so than younger people. Nearly half of the persons questioned in fact said they would prefer to wait an extra day to see their own doctor. It remains to be seen how patients will view this matter after a few years' experience of the centre.

Some Comments on Methods and Future Possibilities

Where does all this get us? The results and methods described all seem rather straightforward, though at the time it seemed that a tremendous amount of effort had to be expended by all concerned to collect and process even this information. The writer is a statistician and very conscious that there is little evidence in this paper of the sophisticated and powerful ways of designing and analysing enquiries which are described in the statistical literature. It seems well worth attempting a simple factorial-type design for an enquiry when two or three new factors are about to be introduced at a site and where their introduction can be effected separately.

The main emphasis in the before-and-after studies described, has been on collecting information about individual consultations with the doctor. Many consultations are multiple in the sense that two or three people are treated simultaneously. Even single consultations often involve somebody's accompanying the sick person. Thus for many purposes it may be more relevant to collect linked information about the little cluster of people involved in the consultation. This method of data collection was tried in study 4 above but it proved difficult to obtain information about the peripheral participants in a consultation. It seems worth trying to persist with this approach using more convenient forms of data-recording stationery, etc. Extending the use of pre-coded records is one partial answer though these can take up a great deal of space especially when one has to make room for a consultation cluster involving a variable number of individuals.

The linking of information longitudinally may also throw further light on the effects of an innovation on the medical care provided,[19] e.g. a more effective method of operation may mean that certain ailments are diagnosed and cured more quickly in terms of number of consultations.

The development of plausible mathematical models can serve at least two purposes:

1. If models of fairly general applicability can be developed, one can concentrate data collection on the inputs and establishment of parameter values for these models and so reduce the labour involved as well as facilitate enquiry design.
2. Such models will enable one to explore theoretically the consequences, on a national or regional scale, of innovations. A certain amount of work has been done in this respect for the hospital services (see, for example, the work of Newell, Feldstein and Bithell) but the community health services appear to have received relatively little attention (but see, for example, Froggatt et al., 1969).

[19] E.g. A. Cartwright, op. cit., has used this approach.

It has been suggested[20] that activity sampling may be a useful and easy way to determine the content of the doctor's work. Instead of an observer appearing at intervals and noting what the doctor was doing at these instants one could, it is thought, provide the doctor with a gadget which bleeped from time to time—the doctor recording what he was doing at each bleep! This approach would indicate how the doctor's time is distributed but not, of course, what he does by way of items of service, etc.

There is probably more room for 'market research' on what people want of a health service and what they think of innovations. There is the delicate problem that such enquiries may sometimes appear to invite criticism of individual health service workers. Even this may be more useful and less painful than it sounds. The writer along with most of his colleagues has had his performance in a number of respects as a lecturer (content, clarity, audibility, mannerisms, etc.) assessed in a survey by his students and found their criticism generous and helpful.

So far one has been talking mostly about specific research projects designed to assess the consequences of innovation. It is arguable, however, that most substantial new developments such as the opening of a health centre should be monitored, at least to the extent of recording some standard basic details of the development and the aspects of life and work likely to be affected by the change (N.B. as observed by the hospital centre in some of their hospital evaluation schemes, this means collecting information before as well as after the setting up of the new development). In this way a great deal of information which at present, if available, tends to be disseminated only in the locality of the new development, might be usable on a much wider scale in the health services.[21]

The comments above emphasise the multi-disciplinary nature of studies of medical care provision. This calls for a sympathetic but not uncritical understanding of one another's skills and approaches, by the representatives of the various disciplines involved in such work. At the moment, people trained in economics and accounting seem to be less in evidence among those working on community health service problems than behavioural scientists and statisticians. Perhaps this conference will repair this apparent deficiency.

[20] C. B. Floyd, 1969 (pers. comm.).
[21] This implies the setting up of some central data-collecting unit.

REFERENCES

Bailey, N. T. J., 'A Study of Queues and Appointment Systems in Hospitals Out-Patient Departments, with Special Reference to Waiting Times', *Journal of the Royal Statistical Society*, Series B, vol. 14, 1952, p. 185.

Beardwood, J., Halton, J. H., and Hammersley, J. M., 'The Shortest Path through many Points', *Proceedings Cambridge Philosophical Society*, vol. 55, 1959, p. 299.

Bevan, J. M., and Draper, G. J., *Appointment Systems in General Practice*, The Nuffield Provincial Hospitals Trust, London 1967 (O.U.P.).

Bithell, J. F., 'The Statistics of Hospital Admission Systems', *Journal of the Royal Statistical Society*, Series C, vol. 18, 1969, p. 119.

Cartwright, A., *Patients and their Doctors*, London 1967 (Routledge and Kegan Paul).

Cox, D. R., and Smith, W. L., *Queues*, London 1961 (Methuen).

Feldstein, M. S., 'A Binary Variable Multiple Regression Method of analysing Factors affecting peri-natal Mortality and other Outcomes of Pregnancy', *Journal of the Royal Statistical Society*, Series A, vol. 129, 1966, p. 61.

Floyd, C. B., 'Car Service in General Practice: A Two-year Survey', *British Medical Journal*, vol. 2, 1968, p. 614.

Froggatt, P., Dudgeon, M. Y., and Merrett, J. D., 'Consultations in General Practice', *British Journal of Preventive & Social Medicine*, vol. 23, 1969, p. 1.

Newell, D. J., 'Statistical Aspects of the Demand for Maternity Beds', *Journal of the Royal Statistical Society*, Series A, vol. 127, 1964, p. 1.

Royal College of General Practitioners, *The Practice Nurse*, Reports from General Practice, No. 10, London 1968.

ACKNOWLEDGEMENTS

It will be clear that the studies described above were the work of many hands. The relevant publications cited list those to whom I owe a debt of gratitude. In the case of studies for which a published report is not yet available the following have between them borne a major part of the burden of designing the enquiries: Dr K. S. Dawes and Dr P. Kay and their colleagues and my colleagues at the University of Kent, especially Mrs E. J. C. Mitchelhill and Miss G. G. Baker. This paper represents a personal view of the work undertaken and I take full responsibility for its shortcomings. The work has been supported by generous grants from the Department of Health and Social Security, the Nuffield Provincial Hospitals Trust and the Nuffield Foundation.

COMMENT ON 'SOME STUDIES OF THE CONSEQUENCES OF REALLOCATION AND RELOCATION OF FUNCTION WITHIN THE COMMUNITY HEALTH SERVICES'

A. L. COCHRANE

Director, Epidemiological Research Unit (South Wales), Medical Research Council, Cardiff

In making some critical comments about these studies, may I first stress how important I believe it to be that sociologists should work in this sphere, how difficult their work is, and how conscious I am that some of their difficulties are due to members of my profession. I can only assure them that they often treat me just as badly!

The first point I want to raise is the medical area in which these studies are centred. If I may be allowed an analogy with medical research, I would like to compare this sort of work with what we call 'phenomenology' in medical circles. This refers to the detailed study of biochemical or physiological mechanisms which are only very vaguely associated with medicine's main problems—the prevention and treatment of disease and the associated social problems. In the same way the sociologists in their studies seem to be studying the epi-phenomena of medicine. They seem almost uninterested in how the reallocation and relocation of functions will affect the efficacy of therapy. They seem over-interested in 'means', and under-interested in 'ends'.

Having said this it is clearly up to me to suggest what I think they ought to be doing and here I have a clear-cut proposal. One of the most urgent areas of medical research at present is the investigation of the importance of the location of treatment and length of stay in hospital. In the first group one has to randomise particular disease groups between hospital, out-patients and home. In the latter one has to randomise the length of stay to find the optimum from the patients' point of view. All such work requires a great deal of sociological and economic assistance, and I feel that such work needs much higher priority.

There are some other points that deserve comment:

1. I cannot agree with the statement on p. 121: 'A controlled experiment even in the limited sense of the clinical or agricultural trial is seldom possible.' I agree that there are areas where randomisation is difficult. There are very many areas where double-blind trials are impossible, but there are very large areas where randomisation is possible and very necessary and for which sociological and economic skills are required. I sometimes feel that sociologists have an inbuilt bias against experimentation, but it may be due to my unfortunate selective experience!
2. If one cannot randomise I agree entirely with all the difficulties mentioned as associated with the interpretation of the results.

Turning now to the individual studies:

(1) *The Appointment System*. Ideally of course one would have liked to see the study conducted on a random sample of doctors, who did not have appointment systems, a random half of whom were persuaded to introduce them; but I am sure everyone will be convinced that appointment systems save waiting time and that most patients and most doctors like them. There is no evidence produced that there is an improvement in medical efficacy. In general I feel that the introduction of appointment systems might be left to natural selection. Some patients will always prefer an 'on demand' system and the number of doctors without appointment systems will probably adjust themselves to the demand. The one point I would like to raise is the cost of this marginal improvement. There does not seem to be enough detail.

(2) *Delegation*. The introduction of para-medical personnel is an important idea. The findings are what might be expected: reduced driving time and increased consultation time. Surely, however, the all-important thing to investigate is the effect on the patients' diagnosis and treatment. I would guess that it would have absolutely no effect, but if one is going to do such an investigation this is surely the most important index. Here again one would like to know more about the cost of giving the doctors more time.

(3) *The Minibus*. This raises similar problems—doctors' time

saved at an undetermined cost with no evidence about the medical effect.

In conclusion, while congratulating Mr Bevan and his colleagues on their hard, accurate work, I should like to return to my original point and suggest that their work would be even more fruitful if they measured purely medical indices as well.

A COST-BENEFIT APPROACH TO MEDICAL CARE*

G. TEELING-SMITH

Director, Office of Health Economics

The Office of Health Economics was created by the pharmaceutical manufacturers in 1962, because of their concern at that time over the widespread misunderstandings about expenditure on health. It was never envisaged that we would do extensive field research, but we have attempted to put into perspective trends in health expenditure, to discuss the factors underlying these trends, and to balance expenditure against the benefits gained from it. This paper reviews the work which we have done in this latter field, and some of the conclusions which we have reached from it.

As far as the costs of sickness and medical care in Britain are concerned, the existence of the National Health Service provides a unique opportunity for their analysis. The direct costs of sickness can generally be readily obtained from published sources. Hospital costs, for example, which account for almost two-thirds of the total expenditure on the NHS, can be analysed from the hospital costing returns and the Hospital In-Patient Enquiry.[1] This analysis gives estimates of the total in-patient costs for different diseases. The only difficulties arise with certain items such as intensive care units, operating theatres and the pharmacy, on which expenditure varies considerably according to the diagnosis but whose costs can only be allocated on a proportionate basis between all patients. These types of cost are relatively small compared with the total running cost of the hospitals, however, and reasonably meaningful figures can be produced for the hospital costs of each type of disease.

The costs of general practice and the medicines prescribed by GPs can also be allocated between diseases.[1] There has been one

---

* This paper was presented by Mr W. Laing, Office of Health Economics.

[1] For detailed discussion of sources and methods of allocating costs of both hospitals and general medical and pharmaceutical services, see Appendix in: Office of Health Economics, *The Costs of Medical Care*, London 1966.

146

major study of morbidity carried out in co-operation between the Registrar General's office and the College of General Practitioners in 1955/56, and this is shortly to be repeated. In addition, market research data are available on a continuing basis from a rotating sample of GPs. Both record the numbers of different diagnoses for which GPs are consulted. Incidentally, there are interesting differences in the diagnostic patterns recorded from these two sources. Both samples are to some extent self-selected. The former were research-minded members of the College, by no means representative of practitioners as a whole. The second, although drawn from a random sample, yield little more than a 50% response rate and, although some checks are carried out on non-respondents, those who co-operate with a market research company may be somewhat non-representative. Presumably as a result of these factors, certain of the more specific and esoteric diagnoses occurred much more frequently in the College report than they do in the market research ones. Again, however, as the diagnoses concerned are relatively infrequent this produces an only marginal effect. Thus, provided one is prepared to take each consultation as having an equal 'cost' one can fairly accurately allocate the total expenditure on the general medical services between diagnoses. The pharmaceutical costs can be allocated even more precisely from market research data, which indicate on the one hand the total sales of each different medicine and on the other the relative numbers of the different diagnoses for which each are prescribed.

Local authorities' costs are more difficult to allocate, as little is known about the cases handled by district nurses, for example. Some estimates can be made, however, of the costs to be allocated to pregnancy and to various immunisation programmes, a point which will be discussed later. Hospital out-patient costs are also not broken down into disease categories and one is left to make estimates based on the breakdown between specialties. Nevertheless it remains true in broad terms that both hospital in-patient costs and the costs of medical care provided in the community can readily be allocated to disease categories.

Days of absence from work due to sickness are directly classified according to the diagnosis written on the absence certificate. These exclude absence of less than three days and certain occupational classes such as the civil service. Apart from this, the numbers of days recorded from each diagnosis can be converted into an economic loss from that cause by multiplying them by the average daily productive contribution of the working population as a whole. This is not, of course, a perfect method because the economic impact of absence will vary substantially between individuals. It does, once again however, give a valid order-of-magnitude figure for the cost of each disease in terms of lost production. As an aside, this is not regarded as true in underdeveloped countries where there is often a massive excess of labour and consequent underemployment. There, unfitness to work is often regarded by governments as involving no economic cost whatsoever.

Real conceptual difficulties start to arise, however, with attempts to quantify losses due to the premature deaths from disease, as recorded in the Registrar General's statistics. The most extreme calculations have assumed that the cost of a premature death should be calculated from the anticipated value of all future production of that individual had he survived to retirement, this figure then being suitably uplifted for the so-called multiplier effect! Although we used somewhat more realistic calculations of the cost of premature mortality in our earliest OHE publications, we now regard even a simple annual value of production lost from current mortality (such as the Americans have used to support their heart and cancer campaigns) to be misleading. The real effect of changes in mortality come in their long-term effect on the demographic structure of the community and these may not always be beneficial. Certainly in some cases reduced mortality can add to costs. In heart disease, for example, we have shown that elimination of deaths from this cause, which predominantly affects the elderly, would over a period of time be expected to add two retired dependants to the population for each active worker saved.[2] Thus while these individuals would enjoy the benefit of a longer life the community as a whole could expect to be no better off.

For the present, we have, therefore, fallen back on the general statement that preventing premature death in young adults should bring short-term economic benefits, while prolonging life among those about to retire probably does the reverse. The eventual effects in either case, however, will be no more than one factor influencing the

[2] See Table H in: Office of Health Economics, *The Common Illness of our Time*, London 1966.

total demographic pattern, which may be much more significantly affected by other factors such as migration and changes in the birth rate. We therefore now exclude any calculations of costs or savings in relation to premature mortality from our discussions.

Over the years, the OHE has undertaken a number of studies to see how costs of various diseases have been reduced by therapeutic progress, and attempted to assess the economic benefits against the cost of achieving them. There are several outstanding examples of substantial savings, e.g. diphtheria, tuberculosis, pneumonia and probably mental illness. We have not in fact studied the first of these because it had passed into history some time before the OHE was established. It was, however, a classic case of a common disease which affected mainly the young being completely controlled by an immunisation programme. In the 1930s it killed about 3,000 children per year; immunisation made it virtually unknown. In such a case, the savings would be expected to be substantial. MacQueen estimated, for example, that in Scotland the introduction of immunisation saved the NHS about £900,000 per year, mainly through a reduction in beds required in isolation hospitals.[3]

The first study which the OHE published was on TB in 1962.[4] This was one of the studies which introduced estimates of production by those who would have died from the disease had the decline in mortality not been accelerated by the introduction of the anti-tubercular compounds (and incidentally overlooked the savings due to reduced sickness absence!). It was not, in general, a very sophisticated piece of economic analysis, but it estimated savings of £40 million per year from reduced mortality and £15 million per year from a reduction in hospital beds. The latter figure was based on the total reduction in numbers of beds occupied by TB patients, between 1952 and 1960. This was probably a correct method as there was a very substantial waiting list for the sanatoria in the early 1950s, so that no reduction in beds could have been foreseen without the chemotherapeutic developments.

We have recently taken a more up-to-date look at the savings from TB. Naturally these are now substantially greater than in 1962, both because of the effects of inflation and rising costs and because of a

[3] MacQueen I. A., *1960 Report of the Medical Officer of Health for Aberdeen*, Aberdeen 1961.

[4] Office of Health Economics, *Progress against Tuberculosis*, London 1962.

further decline in morbidity. Between 1954 and 1967, sickness absence due to respiratory TB fell from 24,660,000 to 4,360,000 days per year. If there had been no such reduction, TB would have cost the National Insurance fund an additional £21 million in sickness benefits last year. In terms of lost production, these £20 million days of sickness absence saved would have cost the country in the region of £75 million last year.[5] In addition, the number of hospital beds occupied by TB patients fell from 21,500 in 1957 to 6,000 in 1967, representing a saving of £30 million per year.[6] For the reasons discussed above, we made no estimate of economic contribution of those whose lives were saved, but it is worth noting that in England and Wales in 1930 there were over 14,000 deaths from TB among those aged 15–29—the age group just starting to contribute to production and national wealth. By 1967 that figure had fallen to 13. Even on this still relatively crude analysis, there can be no doubt that this is a case where the economic savings have overwhelmingly exceeded all the costs of the preventive and therapeutic measures which have accelerated the decline of TB.

Pneumonia is another disease which often affected young people and which also has responded to antibiotic therapy. Work lost through sickness from this cause fell from 1,550,000 days in 1954 to 800,000 days in 1967, representing a saving in production of some £2·8 million per year. The number of hospital beds occupied by pneumonia patients in England and Wales fell from about 4,500 in 1954 to about 3,600 in 1967. This represents a saving of about £2·5 million per year. The mortality pattern for pneumonia is also interesting. This is a case where the trends were downward for all age groups in the first three decades of this century. The introduction of the sulphonamides and antibiotics accelerated the downward trend for the younger age groups, but this was followed by a reversal of the trend for the over 65 age group. Thus in this case therepeutic progress increased the number of young survivors but apparently also in-

[5] This and subsequent calculations assume that an individual's productive contribution is exactly equal to his earnings. Actual production per employee is obviously greater than this, but the difference is assumed to be accounted for by other economic inputs. The number of days of absence are taken from the reports of the Ministry of Social Security (formerly Ministry of Pensions and National Insurance) for the relevant years.

[6] These and subsequent estimates are based on figures for numbers of beds occupied from the hospital In-patient enquiry for the relevant years, and current costs per occupied bed from the hospital costing returns for 1967.

creased the probability of dying from the disease once one had reached retirement. For the oldest age group (the over 75s) the death rates for men in 1956–60 would have been expected to fall to 64% of the 1931–35 rates on the 1901–35 trend. In fact, the 1956–60 rate rose to 182% of the 1931–35 rate.[7] It is nice to think of this as being a case where the antibiotics have merely postponed mortality from this cause until the age of retirement, rather than eliminating it altogether. As one geriatrician put it recently, pneumonia is still the 'old man's friend'. The cost of antibiotics prescribed for pneumonia in the NHS is now some £1·5 million per year. Even assuming that those prescribed for other respiratory infections in order to prevent pneumonia cost as much again, this is another disease where there is a clear-cut economic benefit from recent medical progress.

The last example of this sort is mental illness. In the early 1950s there was a rising trend in the number of beds occupied in mental departments of hospitals. Changes in medical practice which coincided with (and to some extent were made possible by) the introduction of the tranquillisers and anti-depressants, again reversed this trend. The number of occupied hospital beds fell from 151,500 in 1954 to 119,000 in 1968. Taking the average costs for beds in mental hospitals, this fall represents a saving of £24 million per year which can be set against the NHS expenditure of about £16 million per year on psychotrophic medicines. Looking beyond the NHS, however, the reduction in hospital beds has not been accompanied by a corresponding reduction in sickness absence. Over the same period there has been a rise of 8·6 million in the number of days lost from this cause, an increase of about 30%. In terms of lost production this increase would have more than offset the savings in hospital costs.

This is the sort of fact which bedevils cost-benefit studies in this field. On the one hand, one can say that therapeutic progress has achieved nothing in economic trends. The increase in sickness absence may be due to a failure to stem the rising tide of mental illness in terms of getting patients back to work (although it has been possible to get them out of hospital). On the other hand, the rise in sickness absence due to mental illness may be considered in the light of general trends of sickness absence. Most 'minor' diseases have been responsible for

[7] See Table B in: Office of Health Economics, *Pneumonia in Decline*, London 1963.

increasing numbers of absences over the past decade. For some symptomatic diagnoses, absence rates have more than doubled. One is tempted to explain this on the grounds that the public has been more ready to take time off for these minor causes, rather than because the diseases themselves have become more common. The less serious types of mental illness might be among the causes for which this would be true, and hence for which a substantial increase in absence was to be expected. This view is supported by the fact that the greatest increase in absence has been in the 'anxiety' conditions. Thus it is possible that the rise in sickness absence due to mental illness would have been even greater had there been no therapeutic progress in this field. Clearly, however, there must be further study before we can be sure that there has been an overall economic saving from progress against mental disease.

There are other examples where an economic saving for the NHS might have been expected, but where it is doubtful if it has materialised. One such case is poliomyelitis. This was always a relatively rare disease, affecting less than 1,000 persons per year, until the epidemic in 1946 when nearly 8,000 cases were notified. (In an epidemic year, measles affected almost 100 times as many people.) Rather more than half these cases showed some degree of paralysis and some, of course, suffered almost total disability. Nevertheless we have estimated that the cost of treatment and support for individuals, taken together with their own loss of earnings, only exceeds the cost of the polio immunisation campaign if one assumes that the epidemic of the late 1940s and early 1950s would have continued. At the incidence rates of the earlier years, the costs of immunisation exceeded what would have been the total economic cost of the disease. Taking NHS costs alone, immunisation would only have shown an economic payoff if the number of cases had continued to exceed 2,800 per year.[8] In the nature of epidemics it is possible that the incidence would have fallen naturally to below this level.

This calculation was one of the first major blows to our earlier tacit assumption that progress in medical care—and preventive medicine in particular—could normally be assumed to bring economic benefits. No one would suggest on the basis of this analysis, of course, that the polio immunisation campaign should not have been

[8] See: Office of Health Economics, *The Price of Poliomyelitis*, London 1963. The figures are based on 1961 costs.

undertaken. It has helped to explain, however, why expenditure on health has continued to rise despite the conquest of so many diseases.

Recently the OHE has devoted much of its attention to the economic aspects of another form of preventive care: health screening and early diagnosis. The general interest in these subjects has arisen from the very uneven levels of demand for medical care between different individuals if they are left to seek treatment at their own discretion. With the present 'on demand' approach, some people call for medical care frequently and for the most trivial conditions; others fail to seek medical attention for serious and prolonged disorders. The difficulty is exaggerated by the gradual and often insidious onset of many common degenerative diseases, which makes it hard for even the most intelligent to know whether treatment is justified. Screening for early signs or symptoms of serious illness can theoretically provide an alternative approach which is much more likely to select for treatment those who can most benefit from it.

The cost of such a screening programme is affected by at least four factors:

(a) the cost of the screening tests themselves, in terms of equipment, materials and manpower;

(b) the cost of contacting the desired public and ensuring that they attend for examination (this in turn, will depend on the location of the screening, on how comprehensively the population is to be covered and on how many different tests are carried out simultaneously);

(c) the specificity of the tests, i.e. the number of 'false positives' which will subsequently require needless investigation;

(d) the incidence and duration of onset of the disease, which between them determine the frequency with which the same population must be re-screened.

The benefits derived from a screening programme also depend on several factors:

(a) the seriousness of the disease for the individual and the community;

(b) the prevalence of the disease, which will determine the number of cases detected by a given number of examinations;

(c) the sensitivity of the tests, which will determine the proportion of the total number of cases which will be brought to treatment;

(d) by far the most important, the extent to which the prognosis of the disease can be affected by treatment after it is detected—there is no benefit at all (and consequently no purpose in screening) if treatment does not improve the prognosis, or if it is unacceptable to the patient.

Much of the early enthusiasm for health screening derived from its obvious contribution to the conquest of TB. This was a case where a convenient and relatively inexpensive method of mass radiography had been developed shortly before the introduction of the anti-tubercular compounds, such as PAS, streptomycin and isoniazid. The screening of whole populations (e.g. all employees in a particular group of factories) quickly identified those with lung abnormalities which might be indicative of TB. These could be followed up by further examination and confirmed cases could be treated. The number of 'false positives' was relatively small, and in any case positive observations included some other serious conditions such as lung cancer. Effective treatment of practically all detected cases of TB was possible. Most important of all, there was a public health benefit from the early diagnosis of this infectious disease.

Against this background, it was naïvely assumed that corresponding benefits would accrue from similar screening programmes for other diseases. This overlooked three basic considerations:

1. The public health aspect did not arise with chronic but non-communicable diseases such as cancer or diabetes.
2. The natural history of these chronic diseases had never been properly studied. A disease like TB often progressed steadily from a first initial infection by the invading organism to an eventually fatal condition. However, there was no justification for assuming that the same would normally occur in quite different types of disease also.
3. Associated with this, there was often no clear-cut definition of the disease state itself and no hard evidence of whether treatment would improve the prognosis of 'borderline' cases.

Thus early screening programmes yielded many equivocal results and raised more questions than they answered. For this reason, an advisory committee to the OHE in 1966 invited a number of experts to write papers reviewing the medical and economic status of health screening in various diseases. A similar series of studies was also commissioned by the Nuffield Provincial Hospital Trust at about the same time and was published in 1968.[9] Seven of the OHE studies have also now been published and from both series a fairly clear-cut picture has emerged.[10]

High blood pressure provides a good example of the problems, which were summarised in the OHE report by Professor W. W. Holland as follows: 'High blood pressure is not in its own right a common cause of death or of admission to hospital. It is, however, a major factor associated with atherosclerosis and its complications. Arterial blood pressure tends to rise with age; in the sixth decade half of the population have blood pressures which would be defined as "abnormal" by conventional criteria. Those with high blood pressure run a greater risk of mortality than those whose blood pressure is "normal". However, the correlation between blood pressure and mortality is statistical rather than individual. Thus, hypertension as a disease must be defined by the presence of signs and symptoms in conjunction with the pressure level.'[11] Furthermore, this is a typical case where little is known of the natural history of the disease. It has not yet been established how frequently moderately raised levels of blood pressure progress to dangerously high levels, or whether this progression can be halted by therapeutic intervention. Thus the need at present is for good clinical practice, so as to identify cases requiring treatment as much from their symptoms as from their sphynomanometer readings; and at the same time carefully controlled prospective epidemiological studies need to be undertaken in respect of the borderline hypertensive groups.

A very similar picture emerges for a whole range of screening procedures, e.g. haemoglobin measurements for anaemia, blood sugar levels for diabetes and cholesterol for coronary heart disease. A large proportion of the population has 'abnormal' levels, but as yet for most of these the clinical significance for the present or future is

[9] The Nuffield Provincial Hospitals Trust, *Screening in Medical Care. Reviewing the Evidence*, London 1968 (O.U.P.).
[10] The OHE studies published so far cover raised arterial blood pressure, visual defects, cancer of the cervix, depression, ischaemic heart disease, some diseases of the lung and anaemia. *OHE Early Diagnosis Papers*, Nos 1–7, London 1967.
[11] W. W. Holland, 'The Early Diagnosis of Raised Arterial Blood Pressure', *OHE Early Diagnosis Papers*, No. 1, p. 3.

hard to predict in individual terms. Thus one cannot do a cost-benefit equation at present because the benefits are unknown; it is not justifiable on economic grounds to put substantial resources into screening programmes while the epidemiological research needed to assess their value is still in progress. For the present, these sorts of disorder must remain in the field of traditional clinical medicine with the primary responsibility on the GP to detect their presence during his normal doctor-patient contacts. This conclusion was strongly endorsed by a Department of Health and Social Security assessment on the Multiple Health Screening Clinic at Rotherham, which reported that the 'economic effects attributable to the output of the Rotherham clinic in 1966 are proportionately very small. A comprehensive screening system under which he or she were eligible would consume resources equivalent to a major portion of the Rotherham Health Department budget currently available. The cost of following up screened cases (treatment and process after referral) is likely to be a significant multiple of corresponding screening costs—whether of actual or potential clinic output.'[12]

The Department of Health, of course, has some interest in containing expenditure and could, therefore, be expected to view the whole question of early diagnosis with certain reservations. They are perhaps anxious to guard against a repetition of their experience with cervical cytology. In that case, there is a strong presumption that the detection and removal of 'precancerous' cells in the neck of the womb would prevent the subsequent development of clinical cancer of this site, which kills about 2,500 women each year in Britain. The government responded to widespread public demand for a nationwide screening service to reduce this mortality, even though many epidemiologists at the time questioned the assumption on which the demand was based. They have suggested that the 'precancerous' condition may not invariably progress to clinical cancer, and that clinical cases may instead develop after a 'precancerous' phase which is too short-lived to make presymptomatic diagnosis practicable. This still remains an unresolved issue, because the epidemiological evidence from parts of the world such as British Columbia, which has many years' experience of a cervical screening programme, is still open to dispute. One of the greatest problems in

[12] Department of Health and Social Security, *Reports on Public Health and Medical Subjects*, No. 121, London 1969 (H.M.S.O.).

this case has arisen because the lower social classes, who are most at risk from cancer of the cervix, are the least willing to attend screening clinics. This is not only regrettable in personal terms, but also confuses the interpretation of the statistics. At present, therefore, although there remains good reason to expect the screening programme to reduce mortality, there is not yet proof that it will do so. The estimated cost of the screening programme at £3 million per year, together with an increased bed requirement for the treatment of early 'precancerous' cases, therefore still cannot be justified on rigorous scientific grounds. The government would presumably be reluctant to finance other preventive programmes whose benefits were to remain similarly unknown until the assumptions on which they depend had been proved correct. Furthermore, even if the cervix campaign does greatly reduce mortality, it is doubtful if long-term hospital savings would offset the costs of screening. On 1961/62 costs we estimated that a successful five-yearly screening programme would result in a net increase in NHS costs of £300,000 per year.[13]

It is probably true that across the whole range of health screening the introduction of programmes will increase costs to the health services. As OHE has repeatedly said, it is always cheaper for the NHS to allow a patient to die than to seek out his illness and treat it. Furthermore, it is by no means necessarily true that there will be an economic payoff in terms of national production from such programmes. They may well represent a real and very substantial new burden on the national economy. Government must, nevertheless, be prepared for hard epidemiological evidence to come up within the next five or ten years which will prove unequivocally that morbidity and mortality from some diseases *can* be reduced by presymptomatic detection and subsequent corrective medication. Once this happens, public pressure based on sound scientific evidence will demand screening programmes. The economic significance of this is something which government would be well advised to consider in advance.

This brings me to the conclusions we have reached so far in attempting a cost-benefit approach to medical care. There are a few conspicuous and dramatic cases where therapeutic progress has yielded great economic savings to both the NHS and the economy as a whole. It is, surprisingly, probably more difficult to find similar

[13] Office of Health Economics, *Factors which may affect Expenditure on Health*, London 1964.

examples in the field of classical preventive medicine, although diphtheria is certainly one such case. Once one starts to analyse the economic consequences of presymptomatic diagnosis—the searching out of otherwise undetected disorders—it becomes even more difficult to find savings to set against the costs. This is mainly, at present, because the benefits of early diagnosis have not yet been established; it will take long-term, controlled trials to do this. It is probable, however, that even when the clinical benefits are known they will not be accompanied by corresponding economic benefits. Thus one comes back to the inevitable conclusion that the payoff for most medical care comes in personal and social benefits for the individual and his family. Those cases where there has also been a substantial economic benefit for the community as a whole are an exception. The economic savings in these cases are a bonus in addition to the personal benefits of medical care; they cannot be expected to justify expenditure on the health services as a whole.

COMMENT ON 'A COST-BENEFIT APPROACH TO MEDICAL CARE'

J. WISEMAN

Director, Institute of Social and Economic Research, University of York

---

Mr Teeling-Smith's paper provides a survey of actual cost-benefit studies undertaken by the Office of Health Economics, a dispassionate assessment of problems and difficulties, and an identification of some of the outstanding research areas such as preventive medicine and presymptomatic diagnosis.

He is appropriately tentative about the potential practical value of cost-benefit studies in the health field. How, for example, are we to deal with the problem that such studies estimate 'benefit' by calculating the extension of working life expected to result from given health investments, *using the standard life-tables as the basis for calculation*? For cost-benefit studies to influence policy, there must be enough results available to guide not just absolute decisions about the size of the health sector, but also choices between one type of investment (condition) and another. It may be plausible to use existing life-tables for the cost-benefit study of an individual condition. But a fallacy of aggregation clearly enters if the exercise is extended to cover a significant part of health investment. People kept alive by the investments being studied are yet assumed to be dying at the same ages as before! There are statistical techniques available to deal with this but, as Mr Teeling-Smith points out, there is still a long way to go before we are in a position to take advantage of them.

Indeed, perhaps the most valuable question a commentator can ask is: how can cost-benefit studies best be developed in order best to improve policy decisions? (This, it should be emphasised, is not the same question as: how do we get more money for the health service?). The paper suggests three broad areas of interest:

(1) *Past and predictive studies.* Ideally, we would like the latter: what will be the (future) cost-benefit implications of a given programme begun now? But there are no firm statistics about the future:

159

we have no choice but to use historical data. This must frequently be a severe limitation, though of course it is one common to the whole field of human resource studies (how reliable as a *predictor* of the return to a university education being undertaken now are data about the earnings during working life of a graduate of thirty years ago?). The importance of this problem depends upon the particular question we are trying to answer. It is most acute where the incidence of a disabling condition may be long-delayed, its origin difficult to identify and its treatment influenced by innovation. (Attempts to calculate the costs and benefits of screening for TB provide an excellent example.) But there is a general conclusion that is unavoidable: there will always be room for disagreement about the significance of (historic) cost-benefit studies for (future) policy decisions.

(2) *General and incremental studies.* How broad an area must be selected for study, if cost-benefit appraisal is to be policy-relevant? This question clearly has a close affinity with (1). It is tempting to answer it by saying that both have a place, e.g. attempts to assess new and relatively general techniques, and attempts to estimate the consequences of marginal extensions in the use of resources in existing ways for defined purposes. This would be a sufficient answer were research resources not themselves scarce. Paradoxically enough, this scarcity probably argues, in the existing state of knowledge, for a broad rather than a narrow approach, if only because the nature of medical developments has increased the difficulty of narrowly specified studies, at least in some fields (e.g. the incidence of rheumatic fever appears to have declined in the U.K. without any specific attack upon the condition, but rather as a by-product of the use of antibiotics).

(3) *The relation between 'economic' and 'other benefits'.* Historically, cost-benefit studies try to measure 'economic' benefits, in terms of private or community gains in real income from the use of resources to improve health. There is an assumption, usually implicit, that 'economic' benefits can be calculated as a sort of 'starter', 'other' benefits or dis-benefits then being 'added in'. I confess that I am uncomfortable about this procedure. To take but one example, the community stands to gain little or nothing from the devotion of health resources to the treatment of the old. But there is a clear sense in which the community—to say nothing of the old themselves —places a value on such provision. Means must be found to 'weight'

the value to be given to the treatment of the old; this, however, cannot be dealt with simply by an adding-up process, since the whole structure of health *provision* is affected by acceptance of the proposition that services are provided for those who may not produce 'output' but who yet in a real sense derive 'value' from the availability of health services to them.

In my view, there has been much confusion in the discussion of the 'benefits' of health services by economists, deriving essentially from the fact that cost-benefit studies, starting from the analogy of industrial production, identify 'benefit' with 'output' (i.e. improvement in productive capacity), rather than with 'value' (utility to the person treated or the society of which he is a member). The latter may include the former, but is clearly not identical with it. Attempts which are now beginning, to estimate 'utility' in the latter sense by the development of 'social indicators', are of some interest; but it is questionable how far they can get, particularly where market evaluations by individuals remain as completely absent as they are in the U.K.

F

Chapter IV

EFFICIENCY AND PLANNING IN
HOSPITAL CARE

USE OF HOSPITAL COSTS IN PLANNING

J. C. BERESFORD
London School of Hygiene and Tropical Medicine

The national standard hospital costing system which has been developed over recent years, has made available more and better information on hospital costs than ever before. It is therefore particularly unfortunate to find, as yet, that the presentation of these valuable statistics is geared more to accountability than to management and planning. There is an almost nineteenth-century concern for costs per in-patient week rather than for costs per case; similarly, there is a wealth of detail regarding unit costs, but these again with hardly any relation to efficiency in terms of costs per case, which receive barely cursory attention. Costs per in-patient week and costs per unit are still of some significance as indicators of efficient resource use in long-stay hospitals, where the accent is on maintaining the patient more or less permanently rather than on cure and discharge. In short-stay hospitals, however, it is far more logical and meaningful to consider the patient's stay and the cost of curing and discharging him.

A simple analysis relating costs per in-patient week and costs per case to hospital throughput, brings this out (throughput = number of cases per occupied bed per week, i.e. reciprocal throughput × 7 = length of stay in days).

The graph (Fig. 1) shows an analysis of seven hospital regions for larger acute (over 100 beds), mainly acute and partly acute hospitals. Table 1 summarises the trends and characteristics of weekly cost against throughput.

It is immediately apparent from the lower curve (Fig. 1) that costs per in-patient week (C) rise as throughput (t) increases. The relation between weekly costs and throughput for the 114 acute hospitals is a good one ($r = 0.41$) and the linear regression of costs per in-patient week on throughput is

$$C = 33 + 20t$$

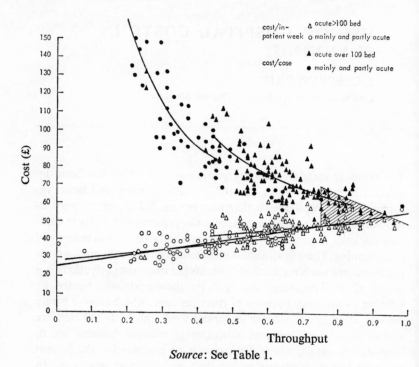

Source: See Table 1.

Figure 1. Hospital Costs on Throughput 1967/68

This may be interpreted as a total cost per in-patient week composed of a weekly hotel, or care and maintenance cost, of £33 and a treatment cost of £20. For example, a hospital with a throughput of 1 would cost £53 per in-patient week; at 0·5, reading from Figure 1, it would cost £43. The mean weighted throughput for the acute hospitals is 0·63 at an average cost of £46 per in-patient week. The 73 mainly acute, and partly acute hospitals yield the regression

$$C = 27 + 22t$$

with a good correlation between weekly costs and throughput ($r = 0·61$). The mean throughput is 0·42 at an average cost of £36·5 per in-patient week. An overall line of best fit for the 187 hospitals ($r = 0·70$) gives the regression

$$C = 26 + 29t$$

The upper curve (Fig. 1) shows the trend for the corresponding

Table 1. Hospital Types: Costs and Throughput 1968

Hospital Type	Costs (C) (£)				Throughput (t)		Correlation of Cost against Throughput	2 Standard Errors on the Regression
	Fixed	Variable		Mean	Mean	Range		
Acute over 100 beds	33·2	20·4t		46·4	0·63	0·44–0·86	0·41	10·81
Mainly and partly acute	27·6	21·9t		36·5	0·42	0·05–0·64	0·61	10·92
Overall line of best fit	26·2	29·5t				0·05–0·86	0·70	9·06

Source: Based on Regional Hospital Board Costing Returns, Parts I–V, for the year ended March 31, 1968.
Note: The ranges include 95% of the hospitals of each type (of the 114 acute hospitals, 3 are excluded below and 3 above the range; of the mainly and partly acute hospitals, 4 are above the range). Some one-third of the variation on the regression is explicable by case-mix differences.

costs per case against throughput. As throughput increases it is evident that costs per case fall, but at a diminishing rate up to about 0·75 throughput. Beyond this, and above 0·8 throughput, the marginal economies of increasing throughput are minimal for the hospitals analysed, the cost per case curve is virtually flat, and at some point, will begin to rise, as negative marginal returns are encountered.

Undue regard for cost per in-patient week is, on this basis, clearly a fallacious indicator of hospital efficiency: the hospitals with heavy costs per in-patient week are also likely to be the least costly hospitals per case treated. The implicit hypothesis is that hospitals giving more intensive treatment, are able to treat and discharge their patients sooner, but that these are likely to incur heavier costs per in-patient week while reducing costs per case. Analysis of the various expenditure categories confirms that expenditure per in-patient week in treatment departments is the most reliable predictor of throughput ($r = 0·46$ overall, range 0·30–0·65).

The fallacy of concentrating on costs per in-patient week can be illustrated further by comparing contrasting regions, such as Liverpool and East Anglia. Liverpool, with a generous allocation of beds per 1,000 of population, is under less pressure and the hospitals in the analysis indicated that it operates at lower throughput and lower cost per in-patient week, but significantly higher cost per case. East Anglia, with a considerably lower bed allocation, spends more per in-patient week but achieves significantly higher throughput and lower costs per case in return. Those kinds of reasons go a long way toward explaining the difference between expenditure at £13·33 per head by the Liverpool Region's hospital services compared with £10·2 per head by the East Anglian Region.

The analysis so far has been extremely simplified but on the other hand a more detailed breakdown of costs into housekeeping and treatment costs is possible as in Table 2, but further analysis along these lines is difficult and may become over-complicated.

The question arises whether there is a theoretical optimum throughput which maximises use of treatment facilities and minimises cost per case. The cross-hatched portion of Figure 1 contains the acute hospitals nearest to optimum throughput and cost per case; they have throughput above 0·75 and the highest is at 0·91 throughput. Cost per week ranges from £40 to £60 and cost per case from £50 to £70. Whereas these are the hospitals nearest to the optimal through-

Table 2. Hospitals Cost per Week Breakdown 1967

Type	Cost per In-Patient Week (£)	Cost Breakdown (£)		
		Wards	Treatment	Other
Teaching London	61·8	22·7	12·8	26·3
Teaching provincial	54·8	20·3	12·9	21·6
Acute over 100 beds	43·6	17·8	7·5	18·2
Acute 51–100 beds	45·5	20·4	6·0	19·1
Acute 1–50 beds	36·7	19·3	3·0	14·5
All acute	43·1	18·2	7·0	17·9
Mainly acute	37·9	16·5	5·1	16·3
Partly acute	31·3	14·4	3·2	13·7
Mainly long-stay	26·6	13·3	1·3	12·0
Long-stay	20·5	10·0	0·6	9·9
Chronic	18·3	9·7	0·2	8·4
Rehabilitation	18·2	4·5	2·4	11·3
Mental subnormality	11·6	4·8	0·5	6·3

Source: See Table 1.

put and cost per case of those analysed, the theoretical optimum for a highly intensive, high-throughput hospital may be even higher.

An acute hospital, and even more so a super-acute hospital, like any productive organisation, is efficient only if its treatment facilities are used intensively during the stay of each patient. A high-tempo, acute or super-acute hospital should be interpreted as one with both relatively high throughput and intensive use of treatment facilities. This is best achieved with a certain amount of specialisation and concentration on a limited number of departments to avoid, where possible, the mixing of short-stay, intensive users of facilities and longer-stay, light users.

On a broader strategic level, if it is accepted that high-tempo, acute hospitals are desirable, treating patients intensively at a high weekly cost but maintaining high facility use and throughput to give lower costs per case, then a new vista of alternatives is opened up. Such a hospital would selectively admit acute patient groups needing intensive treatment and it would operate on progressive care principles moving patients within, and out from, the high-tempo, acute hospital to accommodation appropriate to their care requirements, during their hospital stay. It would also attempt to maintain as high a bed occupancy as possible. Here again, accurate knowledge of facility utilisation and dependency profiles of different patient groups is necessary and suggests considerable scope and potential returns from research in this area.

Perhaps the simplest way of demonstrating the potential of a high-cost, high-tempo, acute hospital is by a hypothetical example. Assume that a common catchment area is served by two general hospitals providing a total of 1,000 beds, each operating at a below-average throughput of 0·55 (= average stay of 12·7 days). Such a length of stay is given by the length-of-stay distribution table, columns one and two, based on the Hospital In-Patient Enquiry, excluding stays over three months (Table 3).

Table 3. Length-of-Stay Distribution

Length of Stay	Number of Discharges	Subgroup of Frequencies	
		Low Average Length of Stay	High Average Length of Stay
Days:			
0–3	105	90	15
4–7	90	80	10
8–14	106	85	21
15–29	64	40	24
Months:			
1–1·9	27	5	22
2–3	8	0	8
Total	400	300	100
Average length of stay	12·7 days	8·9 days	24·1 days

Source: Based on *Hospital In-Patient Enquiry*, 1966.

In columns three and four these frequencies have been arbitrarily divided between two subgroups forming two of the many other possible distributions. Here the 400 discharges of average stay 12·7 days have been divided into a sub-group of 300 discharges with a relatively lower length of stay, 8·9 days—in which five patients stay over one month and none over two months—and another subgroup of 100 discharges with a heavier load of longer-stay patients, producing an average length of stay of 24·1 days.

Suppose two general hospitals, each operating at 0·55 throughput, treat this kind of case load without selecting between long- and

Table 4. Hypothetical Example

Strategy I: No Selection: Hospitals A and B at Below-average Throughput (0·55)

Hospital	Throughput	Beds	Discharges		Cost (£)		
			Per Week	Per Year	Per Week	Per Case	Per Year
A	0·55	600	330	17,160	44.4	80·4	1,379,664
B	0·55	400	220	11,440	44·4	80·4	919,776
		1,000	550	28,600			2,299,440

Strategy II: Selection: Hospital A at High Throughput (0·78), Hospital B at Low Throughput (0·29)

Hospital	Throughput	Beds	Discharges		Cost (£)		
			Per Week	Per Year	Per Week	Per Case	Per Year
(a) A	0·78	529	413	21,476	49·1	62·9	1,350,840
B	0·29	471	137	7,124	34·0	117·2	834,933
		1,000	550	28,600			2,185,773
(b) A	0·90	459	413	21,476	51·6	57·3	1,230,575
B	0·29	471	137	7,124	34·0	117·2	834,933
		930	550	28,600			2,065,550

Note: The number of beds in Strategies II (a) and (b) are obtained from discharges at the set throughput.
0·55 throughput = average stay 12·7 days; 0·78 throughput = average stay 8·9 days; 0·29 throughput = average stay 24·1 days; 0·90 throughput = average stay 7·7 days.

short-stay cases; the results are summarised under Strategy I in Table 4, the total number of discharges being 28,600 at an annual expenditure of £2,299,440. If now selection is introduced and the three-quarters of the case load with a lower average stay (8·9 days) go to hospital A and the other quarter of the case load with a high average stay (24·1 days) go to hospital B, then a different pattern emerges. Strategy II(a) of Table 4 represents a saving of £113,667, i.e. some 5% against Strategy I. However if, as is likely, the high-acute hospital A were able to improve throughput from 0·78 to say 0·90 because of its more intensive treatment, the situation would be shown at Strategy II(b) with a saving of £233,890, i.e. 10% against Strategy I.

These hypothetical examples are meant as illustrations of alternative planning strategies and their implications, rather than as practical estimates of relative saving. As such they are very much simplified. It is not intended to suggest that the patient's length of stay is all that distinguishes the high-tempo, acute hospital; the main criterion is the intensive use of service. Likewise, it is not proposed that there be only two hospital types, one very high-tempo acute, and the other very low-tempo; there would obviously be intermediate types of hospital.

However, the above examples serve to show the potential of a new look at hospital costs with the accent on strategy and planning implications, rather than on costliness as such. The orientation here has been toward fitting care more accurately to need. Two suggestions have been proposed: one is for progressive patient care, even at a relatively crude level, but on a systematic basis which includes staffing and planning of facilities; the other is for a greater accent on high-cost and high-tempo hospitals offering more intensive treatment during a shorter stay.

The case being put is for more precise definition of what a hospital, of whatever type, is meant to provide and for an examination of what it does in fact provide and of the consequences. At present there is a wide disparity between stated definitions and objectives, and actual practice. Hospital-type definitions are often extremely misleading, a fact which requires no elaboration when it is considered that up to one-third of patients in acute accommodation do not need this level of care.

Any practical action on the lines suggested still poses questions of considerable importance. Exactly how high-tempo hospitals should relate to the system is not at all certain, because the whole issue of catchment areas and accessibility arises, which will require further research if any radical changes are planned. Any system which pre-selects patients for different levels of care, threatens the possibility of actual or apparent inequity of treatment; fears on these grounds are very real. Indeed, it may be anticipated that were hospitals to be classified on a relatively strict scale of care provided, the lower categories would encounter considerable staffing and morale problems, and some means would have to be devised of ensuring this did not happen.

All the discussion, thus far, has concerned the whole-hospital situation with regard to throughput and resource consumption, hence its cost. All the cost analysis is made difficult by differences in case-mix of different hospitals. The importance of the case cost has been emphasised, but this was with reference to the average case, and yet there is probably difference in cost between cases in different specialties or in different diagnostic groups. Detailed studies of these differences provide guides to the planning and allocation of facilities, and elaboration on such studies to include an assessment of outcome of treatment would enable a first attempt at resource allocation by cost-effectiveness methods.

Our unit obtained some of the basic information needed for this type of analysis in a research study partially completed this summer. In that study, two of the departmental resources, namely pathology and X-ray facilities, were studied to determine their utilisation by in-patients by diagnostic groups. Eight large, acute hospitals were visited and case notes perused in order to find the pathology and X-ray weighted units consumed by samples of cases in each of some twenty diagnostic groups in both medical and surgical specialties. The prime objective of the study was an attempt to obtain planning estimates of resource use, that allowed for case-mix differences between hospitals. However, the results of this study revealed such large differences in use between hospitals that it is doubtful whether this objective will be achieved fully even with a large increase in the sample sizes. But partial allowance for case-mix can be made by allowing for predominance of diagnostic groups that are heavy or light users of these services and such groups have been identified and are shown in Table 5.

The data are also useful to indicate the cost differences arising in different cases through the differences in the use made of these particular facilities. The next step is to extend this type of study to include the larger cost items of theatre use and nursing man-hours

Table 5. Consumption of Pathology and X-Ray Services by Selected Diagnostic Groups

Diagnostic Group	Weighted Units per Day Pathology	X-ray	Diagnostic Group
High Use			
Hyperplasia of prostate	5·203	0·404	Peptic ulcer
Peptic ulcer	4·545	0·232	Hyperplasia of prostate
Chronic bronchitis	4·025	0·222	Cancer, colon
Weighted mean	4·626	0·229	Weighted mean
Medium Use			
Cancer, colon	3·307	0·185	Pneumonia
Pneumonia	3·148	0·126	Fractured femur
Asthma (children)	3·039	0·123	Cancer, breast
Coronary	3·379	0·111	Asthma
Cancer, cervix	2·449	0·101	CUA
Appendicitis	2·393		
Uterine prolapse	2·215		
Cancer, breast	2·128		
Weighted mean	2·790	0·124	Weighted mean
Low Use			
Fractured femur	0·938	0·093	Cancer, cervix
CUA	1·734	0·094	Chronic bronchitis
Hernia	1·581	0·079	Appendicitis
Varicose veins	0·463	0·077	Hernia
		0·064	Coronary
		0·033	Uterine prolapse
		0·029	Varicose veins
Weighted mean	1·314	0·068	Weighted mean

consumed. Studies of this type are extremely time-consuming and rather difficult to complete and are indicative of the extreme difficulty of introducing a rational basis of planning health services.

Tables 6 and 7 show a selection of case costs and their differences.

Table 6. In-Patient Use and Cost of Pathology and X-ray Services for High-, Medium- and Low-User Diagnostic Groups

	Use by Diagnostic Groups			Cost (£) per Unit
	High	Medium	Low	
Pathology units per day	4·63	2·79	1·31	0·172
X-ray units per day	0·23	0·12	0·07	0·618
Pathology cost (£) per day	0·80	0·48	0·23	
Pathology cost (£) per week	5·60	3·36	1·61	
X-ray cost (£) per day	0·14	0·07	0·04	
X-ray cost (£) per week	0·98	0·49	0·28	

Table 7. Difference in Cost of Surgical and Non-Surgical Cases

	Average Weekly Hospital Cost per Bed (£)
Acute hospitals over 100 beds	46·41
Operating theatre component	5·04
Non-surgical case	41·37
Surgical case, 1 in 3 beds surgical	56·49
Surgical case, 1 in 4 beds surgical	61·53

If outcome were known, and measures of outcome developed, then priority for hospital treatment of different illnesses might be attempted. There is also the question of hospitalisation versus non-hospitalisation, and this decision also requires knowledge of the outcome to cost ratio of hospital versus community care treatment. Although at the present time there are evident attempts to reduce hospitalisation and to encourage community care, little is known about the relative cost or effectiveness of these courses of action.

Even if only direct costs were included, it could be argued that on economic grounds present provision is at a very flat portion of the total cost curve of community and institutional care. Community costs are liable to show an accelerating increase following reduced hospitalisation, whether this results from rapid discharge or non-hospitalisation, on assuming a steady level of quality of care. There is perhaps more scope for economic manipulation within the structure of institutional care itself. There may be administrative charges necessary that would encourage more sensible decisions to be made about the method and place of treatment of the sick person.

Purely on the level of care required and offered in the community and in hospital, our research unit has recently started a study which looks at samples of potential hospital cases when they are being cared for in the community, and at a sample of low nursing dependency cases actually in hospital; a comparison of their circumstances and treatment is being attempted.

Information is available, and is being slowly publicised, showing large differences in health care provision per head of population in different areas. Present data only allows easy comparison on a regional basis, and hospital service expenditure per head of population varies from £9 to over £16 per head in different regions. There is a strong case for more attention to be given to area population denominators in planning, financing and evaluating health care services.

COMMENT ON 'USE OF HOSPITAL COSTS IN PLANNING'

D. J. NEWELL

University of Newcastle Upon Tyne

I begin by briefly summarising Mr Beresford's argument. Hospital-costing schemes are now geared to accountability rather than to management and planning. He shows how a simple expression of cost per case rather than per in-patient week can be helpful. Cost per in-patient week rises linearly with the throughput, but cost per case decreases (perhaps in a parabola) with rising throughput, until the curve flattens out at a throughput of 0·75 patients per occupied bed per week, or an average stay of about 9 days.

From these figures, he suggests that if two unselective hospitals are replaced by a high-throughput and a low-throughput hospital, then a reduction in hospital costs will be achieved. This flies in the face of the concept of all hospitals being general hospitals, and deserves careful consideration. I think the implication is that the unselective hospital may provide facilities for every patient which are used only for a proportion of them—in fact they are assumed to be used mainly by the high-throughput hospital's type of patients. One point not made by Mr Beresford is that his two types of hospital need not be on different sites—the same argument could be applied to sensible differentiation of function within the same hospital—and his separation of the two types of patient could well be replaced, perhaps with even greater efficiency, by the separation of each patient's stay into segments requiring more or less facilities—in other words the progressive patient care concept.

To digress for a moment, I should like to mention the pre-discharge ward. Without going into detail, this is a device to reduce the effect of the stochastic nature of the hospital process: a variable number of patients is admitted each day and their durations of stay are variable. This necessarily means that some beds must be left empty each day. The pre-discharge ward can accommodate patients of either sex, medical or surgical, for the last few days of their stay. As well as being a part of progressive patient care, it does mean a pooling of resources, and thus achieves economies of scale. The important thing from our point of view is that, viewed by itself, the pre-discharge ward is very expensive, as it ideally gathers together all of the variability in bed use, leaving the other wards to remain completely full. So it is misleading to evaluate the parts unless they are related to the whole.

This brings us back to Beresford's paper—the costs of his two hospitals only make sense when they are added together. This principle should really be extended to the whole health service. The expenditure on care outside the hospital should be taken into account where early discharge or out-patient treatment reduces the cost per case within the hospital; even more difficult to take into account is the cost of preventive services—to specify just two, the chiropody service, which helps to keep old people mobile and thus reduces the morbidity due to immobility, and the treatment of incontinence, which quite often seems to be the determinant of whether a family can cope with its elderly patients at home. These costs should be balanced against the saving in hospital expense. The most important thing which Mr Beresford's paper does is to demonstrate the very useful results which can be achieved by very simple analysis of existing data. But we must beware of over-reliance on any single criterion of hospital efficiency. An often-quoted over-reliance on the percentage occupancy illustrates this point. A surgical department criticised for its low occupancy can continue to do exactly the same operations as before, but keep the patients in hospital until the next batch of patients for cold surgery is admitted.

Similarly, Beresford's cost per case could be minimised in theory by allowing patients to die as soon as they had been through the admission procedure; the same result of a low cost per case can also be achieved by admitting patients who do not really require admission, and whose care does not involve expensive procedures or necessarily long durations of stay.

DECISION-MAKING WITHIN HOSPITALS

G. M. LUCK
Institute for Operational Research

INTRODUCTION

My paper consists of three parts: first, some introductory comments on my understanding of the economics of medical care; second, comments on two case studies we have undertaken at hospital and hospital management committee level with particular reference to the economic aspects; and third, comments on the relation of operational research and economics and how they can be used.

I believe that it is relevant to split the economics of medical care into two distinct levels: macro- and micro-economic decisions. The first level includes decisions taken at the national level such as what financial and manpower resources shall be permitted for the National Health Service and how these resources are to be distributed between regions and parts of the NHS. Since we have not been asked to work at this level I cannot be sure that such decisions are taken explicitly, but I shall assume that they must be and shall ask at the end whether our work is likely to have any relevance for them.

In this country the NHS is the principal provider of medical care. The top decision-makers may be more concerned with problems of survival and adaptability than with economic efficiency. By its very existence as a perceived central provider, the NHS acts as 'them' against whom consumers and employees can complain. The NHS may be in unstable equilibrium before these external and internal pressures. Adaptability is necessary because the provision of medical care has so far existed as a largely open system, with new ideas being freely propagated through the professional journals, conferences, etc. This must pose extraordinary headaches for the central decision-makers and their economic advisers.

What I am trying to suggest here is that to some extent morale, survival, adaptability and leadership are important factors in the highest-level decision-making and that economics must compete. I suggest that this also occurs in military fields and industry, two other areas where both economics and operational research have been used.

In the second level, the 'micro-economic', I would include decisions at the hospital and in general practice which affect the day-to-day provision of medical care to patients. In the second part of this paper I shall be referring to work in the hospital field. In the same way as I have hypothesised for the 'macro-decisions', we shall want to consider the factors which are involved in these decisions and how much economics can and does enter into them. I shall assume that any economic model must consist of three components: an input of resources; an output of medical care; and management and organisation which bring the two together more or less efficiently.

CASE STUDIES

Until recently most of our programme of health research[1] has been in the area which we have called 'operational policies'. By this we mean those decisions which are one stage removed from the immediate personal decisions of a doctor and a patient but which directly affect the deployment of resources for such personal decisions. Operational policies are decisions about decisions. The term has been used most often by others to describe decisions made at the stage of a new hospital building when the architect is being briefed. We would contend that operational policies are needed as part of the hospital management process both during building and commissioning, and during operations. They may not, of course, be explicit.

One such study was concerned with the commissioning of a new acute, 600+ bed hospital near Coventry. It was the largest new project in the Birmingham Region, and has been designed for progressive patient care. The board asked us to help develop the policies and take account of the capital and current costs making it necessary to run the hospital at high intensity.

Feldstein[2] has suggested that the potential economies of scale are not achieved in larger hospitals 'primarily due to the lower case-

---

[1] Supported by the Department of Health and Social Security, regional boards and boards of governors.

[2] M. S. Feldstein, *Economic Analysis for Health Service Efficiency*, Amsterdam 1967, p. 86 (North-Holland).

bed ratio in larger hospitals . . . (which) probably reflects a lower level of "managerial" or labour efficiency and, in particular, a slower hospital pace'. The work of my colleagues[3] has suggested that larger managerial units in larger hospitals have the capability of being more efficient, mainly because it is easier to deal with variable admissions.

Direct examination of the cost headings and experience with setting up the policies, show that the short-term variable costs are few. The revenue costs—i.e. excluding capital—I have split into three groups somewhat arbitrarily: non-patient (30%), patient occupancy (24%) and patient treatment (46%). Of the treatment costs, only a small proportion, drugs and dressings, are truly variable, the remainder being principally staff costs which are not variable (although there may be some overtime in treatment departments).

The average costs for three regional hospital boards (RHB) for all acute hospitals over 100 beds[4] are shown in Table 1 together with the estimates for Walsgrave Hospital, first full year, and for the Coventry and Warwickshire Hospital, 1967.

Table 1. Average Cost for Acute Hospitals

	L Non-Patient Cost per Staffed Bed (£)	M Patient Occupancy Cost per Occupied Bed (£)	N Patient Treatment Cost per In-Patient Case (£)
Newcastle RHB	10·31	8·68	41·29
Leeds RHB	10·44	9·58	33·69
Birmingham RHB	11·28	9·60	34·80
Coventry and Warwickshire Hospital	11·08	11·84	30·94
Walsgrave Hospital (estimated)	15·15	16·43	24·86

[3] J. Luckman *et al.*, *Management Policies for Large Ward Units*, Institute for Operational Research Health Report No. 1, London 1969.

[4] Department of Health and Social Security, *Hospital Costing Returns*, Year ended March 31, 1968 (H.M.S.O.).

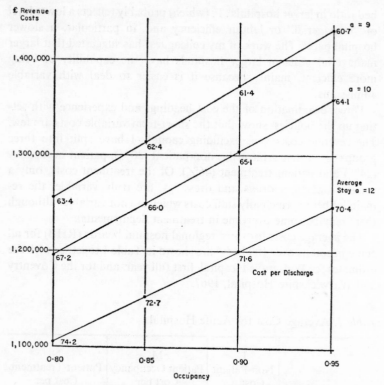

Figure 1. Hospital Costs Related to Stay and Occupancy

The graph (Fig. 1) shows the estimated total cost and cost per discharge for various occupancies and average lengths of stay. It would appear that by increasing certain resources and management efficiency we could put the occupancy up to 90%, so that the total current cost would increase by £50,000 but the cost per discharge decrease by £0·9. The economic answer to this might be:

1. There is no more money available.
2. You can have the extra £50,000 because the cost per discharge is reduced and you are benefiting the community by treating more patients at a lower average cost.
3. The increase is only worthwhile if you can show a compensatory saving elsewhere in the group. We must shut down completely or

partially another hospital in the group, and those patients will make up the increase at Walsgrave.

The increase in number of discharges would be about equivalent to the throughput of a thirty-bed ward. Therefore if this could allow closing a ward in another hospital with a cut in costs including the fixed costs, it would seem worthwhile.

We have considered some of the ways of trying to achieve this efficiency as follows:

(a) scheduling of admissions, predicting occupancy, etc.—an 'information room' has been set up;
(b) a timetable of operating sessions which balances resources—a computer simulation has been used to help set this up;
(c) pre-admission tests of patients from the waiting-list to reduce stay, especially pre-operative, and prevent admission of patients unfit for operation; and
(d) extended working day and week for the hospital (not for staff), e.g. operating sessions at weekends.

It is this latter problem which I have suggested elsewhere could be worth a major initiative.[5] It could help to achieve and surpass the targets in terms of cost per case but, more important, it could give better return on capital which will become increasingly important for the large, new, district general hospitals being planned and built.

We can spend a lot of effort trying to squeeze out a few per cent improvement. However, it may be that greater improvements could be achieved through reconsidering the existing daily and weekly cycles of the hospital. For example, the utilisation of X-ray equipment and staff is very much constrained by the availability of the patient (affected by ward organisation), of porters and of radiologists and radiographers. This usually leads to a quite short period of high activity.[6]

I suggest that we need to try out a hospital 'Fawley'[7] productivity agreement making better use of evenings and weekends. This would

[5] G. M. Luck, 'Three Approaches to Decision-Taking in Hospitals', in: M. E. Abrams (ed.), *Medical Computing: Progress Problems*, London 1970 (Chatto and Windus).

[6] The Nuffield Provincial Hospitals Trust, *Towards a Clearer View*, London 1962 (O.U.P.).

[7] A. Flanders, *The Fawley Productivity Agreement*, London 1960 (Faber & Faber).

reduce much of the slack which now decouples successive daily and weekly pressures. It would be in this situation that a computer would be more important for processing information and scheduling workloads.

In the Walsgrave case study we focussed on the problems of one hospital, deliberately ignoring other related hospitals. In a second case study we were required to examine the short-term reorganisation within a group. There were two main areas of choice: whether to close one of two casualty departments at opposite ends of the group; and how to allocate sixty-five new beds to be opened shortly in one of the four main hospitals of the group. I think that this may be the appropriate place to mention the attempts being made to involve hospital doctors in hospital management started off by the 'Cogwheel Report'.[8] Among the conclusions were:

'(c) The hospital sector is the most costly element of the National Health Service and its use of resources would be improved if its base of activity were wider than the individual hospital.

(e) Within the hospital there is a need for a representative group of clinicians aided as appropriate by operational research to undertake a continuous review of hospital activity, to take an active part in the co-ordination and planning of services . . .'

This project was intended to work on the lines of conclusions (c) and (e).

Our work led to the following preliminary recommendations:

1. Reorganisation should be looked at as a group problem, not as separate hospital problems.
2. The reorganisation should produce a unified medical, nursing and administrative management for hospitals, A and B together, and hospitals C and D together.
3. The regional board and management committee should accept some capital and revenue costs for improved secretarial, statistical and communication services.

Finally, four alternative plans for reallocation of beds were presented for choice. We called these: (i) no change, (ii) marginal solution I, (iii) marginal solution II, and (iv) radical solution.

[8] First Report of the Joint Working Party on the Organisation of Medical Work in Hospitals, London 1967 (H.M.S.O.).

Although economically most attractive, the radical solution would have required reallocation of consultant sessions and closing one casualty department. Both of these were unacceptable.

In reaching the solutions we considered the evidence of internal pressure on specialties in terms of occupancy of beds, the ratio of emergency to planned admissions, and average time on the waiting-list. We also took account of the catchment areas which the specialties were serving. This assumed that the referral process was efficient in the sense that it did not allow admission of a distant patient to displace a nearer patient who was more ill.

In seeking for alternative allocations we devised a simple systematic method which took account of beds and theatre sessions for each specialty, and then generated alternative rearrangements consistent with the available beds and theatre sessions at each of the four hospitals.

In a direct sense then we did not consider the financial costs of any rearrangement, but we did consider the efficiency in terms of patient throughput. The solutions had to be discussed and agreed at open session of the group medical committee. A certain amount of bargaining therefore ensued between consultants in different specialties. Reallocation of consultant sessions usually takes place only on death or retirement and it is therefore not easy to see how positive central direction of hospital medical care can take place.

COMMENTS

I have mentioned briefly two of a number of projects we have undertaken. These have been mainly centred on hospitals—admittedly the most expensive arm of the service—but we are now undertaking projects in area health planning. The hospital studies have suggested that it is possible to produce rather more systematic decision-making in hospitals which does take account of availability of resources, although is less prepared to be explicit about outcomes of health care. A very considerable amount of effort has to go into the discussion and implementation of such changes due to the large number of decision-makers and their lack of familiarity with management thinking. This may improve with spread of ideas through training, courses, professional literature, etc.

Our experience ought to be of value since we are beginning to develop models of hospital activity which should provide information for central decision-makers. I think that we are beginning to advance from the position mentioned by Feldstein:[9] 'Too little is known about the behavioural characteristics of hospital production for us to be certain that any particular (stochastic) specification is the correct one.'

Still thinking at the micro-economic level, two key areas seem to us to need more work. One we have called the 'referral network', which is the sum of the processes and reasons by which people come in contact with and are routed through the health care system. It is fairly clear that this is affected by individual, socio-economic and cultural characteristics but more needs to be known. This is an area into which we are entering.

The second key area is the follow-up of the outcomes of medical care, e.g. the relative value of hospital and home treatment for coronaries. We were asked to do this by the Coventry physicians but decided that our manpower resources were not sufficient and that we did not have the epidemiological skills. To this end, we are now developing a relationship with the Department of Social Medicine at St Thomas' Hospital.

[9] M. S. Feldstein, *op. cit.*

COMMENT ON 'DECISION-MAKING WITHIN HOSPITALS'

V. CARSTAIRS

Scottish Home and Health Department

Mr Luck's paper is about the role of operational research in providing information on which rational decisions can be made about the allocation of resources within hospital, and in the development of management techniques to ensure that the efficient use of resources is maintained.

Undoubtedly, hospitals could be run more efficiently (i.e. consume fewer resources for a given output), and the patient costs given in Mr Luck's paper suggest that this is being achieved at Walsgrave, by 'running the hospital at high intensity'—i.e., I assume, by keeping occupancy high and duration of stay low. He mentions Martin Feldstein's observation that potential economies of scale are not achieved in larger hospitals. As large hospitals are built primarily with the intention of benefiting from economies of scale, it might be useful if the economists could throw some light on the reasons these are not achieved, if this is in fact the case.

Operational research, by suggesting alternative courses of action, can lead to greater efficiency. I believe that operation techniques are making a very considerable contribution in this particular situation and that some of the findings may be relevant to a wider field, although one of the possible drawbacks of operational research solutions is that usually they apply to very specific problems and situations.

Despite the title of his paper, Mr Luck does not say anything much about decision-making and this is a field I should like to move into, from the point of view of considering how decision-making at the within-hospital level may be influenced.

He does say that a considerable amount of effort has to go into the discussion and implementation of such changes 'due to the large number of decision-makers and their lack of familiarity with management thinking'. By and large, consultants are not prompted by considerations relating to the efficient use of resources and are not aware that they are acting in a managerial capacity in laying claim to and disposing of health service resources. There are mechanisms built into the training and the commitment to professional objectives which largely ensure that quality of care for the patient is maintained. Sanctions also exist which are sometimes invoked in cases of malpractice. No such mechanisms or sanctions exist in respect of efficiency.

Most doctors are motivated by the desire to provide excellent treatment for their patients and some by the desire to achieve eminence in their profession. The decisions they take may be seen mainly against this background. The organisational structure of the hospital system has not in the past favoured the pursuit of objectives for the hospital or for the community, but rather the pursuit of objectives as perceived by individual consultants. One of the aims of the reorganisation of medical staff as proposed in the 'Cogwheel Report' is to overcome this proliferation of interests. In this report it is proposed that consultants should group themselves together into divisions based on clinical interest. Among the functions of these divisions would be the maintenance of standards of care, and the pursuit of the management role in the discussion of priorities for the allocation of resources within the hospital.

Within the context of this reorganised structure I should like to raise the question of the content of routine information systems (rather than *ad hoc* studies of the kind described by Mr Luck) which are designed to aid the divisions in the pursuit of the two aims I have described, one of which is concerned with input and the other with output.

In this field of information systems we have some experience, but we are very aware that we have not yet found the right formula. For the first time this year the Scottish Home and Health Department has sent out to all consultants in Scotland a short statistical statement on the patients treated by the consultant, and comparative data for consultants in the same specialty, in the region and in Scotland. We hope that this return will develop into a useful management tool, but perhaps the economists could help in deciding what information relating to efficient use of resources and effective performance, should go into such a return. In the first category our return presently contains information relating to length of stay, and to time spent on the waiting-list. I have suggested, as others have, that cost per case would also be a meaningful measure, but in view of the fact that many costs are outside the immediate influence of the consultant, is this really of any merit (leaving aside the fact that individual patient costs are not in any case available)? Is it possible perhaps to isolate a cost factor which could be attributed to an individual consultant, or would this correlate so highly with length of stay that it would be pointless to produce it? I should mention that information on consultants does not identify the beds at his disposal (a system the service is trying to move away from) so that there is no possibility of measuring efficiency in terms of throughput per bed. In terms of output we have even further to go. Mortality in hospital is now so rare for most conditions that it is no longer a measure of competence. Professional competence is probably judged to a large extent these days by whether the clinician can be seen to have used appropriate methods of investigation and treatment, rather than by the condition of the patient. It seems likely that most of the indices of patient condition that might be developed would involve professional judgements and might be difficult to make operational. In any event, the condition of the patient on discharge may not be a very adequate guide to performance and it seems important that clinicians should be informed about the subsequent course of events. In some cases this happens by attendance at out-patients, but a study was reported from the Oxford Region which enquired into the deaths of patients after discharge: many consultants were surprised to be told that a patient had subsequently died. His ability to assess performance must surely be adversely affected in the absence of such information. While death is an undisputable event, return to work can be affected by many considerations such as the willingness of the GP to tolerate the patient's clinging to the sick role.

How one sells these ideas to consultants is a considerable problem, as feedback from our own enquiry suggested that the one thing consultants do not want to hear about is waiting-list times and duration of stay.

THE IMPLICIT VALUATION OF FORMS OF HOSPITAL TREATMENT

R. J. LAVERS

Institute of Social and Economic Research, University of York

INTRODUCTION AND BACKGROUND

The chief aim of this paper is to examine the possibility of drawing inferences about the relative value placed on the treatment of patients for particular disorders, from a knowledge of the decisions actually made in the hospital system. Interest will thus be focussed on such questions as: Is the treatment in hospital of a peptic ulcer considered to be of greater or less importance than the treatment of varicose veins? Does greater or less value attach to a herniorrhaphy for a young and otherwise able-bodied male than to a hysterectomy for a middle-aged female? Or is one only entitled to say that decision-makers in the hospital service are indifferent between such alternatives? Such questions are held to be of importance because resources in the health service are not unlimited relative to the uses to which they may be put, and therefore choices, whether conscious and explicit or not, continually require to be made. It is thus a matter of some importance to consider, for example, whether the choices currently being made may be improved upon, or whether there exist any inconsistencies in the pattern of choices made (in the sense that, in a given set of circumstances, course of action A appears to be preferred to B, B preferred to C, yet C preferred to A). Not infrequently, of course, decisions about the numbers and types of patients to be treated in hospitals are explicitly revised in the light of further information and after some reflection on priorities: a recent example is provided by the hospital management committee which announced that it had been admitting too many patients for abortions at the expense of an increase in the waiting time and size of waiting-list for gynaecology cases (see *The Times*, July 31, 1969). It is likely that there exists considerable unrecognised scope for such revisions, which presumably modify the health service in such a way that its operation is made more consonant with society's preferences, at national and regional as well as local levels.

One approach that might be adopted in dealing with the problem of improving the mixture of facilities provided in a health service is to posit a value that attaches to each type and scale of facility and to assume a form in which the total mixture of facilities is related to the total value of that mixture. An alternative formulation is to identify and attach 'disvalues' to all the health problems that exist to be solved and assume a form in which the total mixture of problems is related to the total cost of ill-health.[1] The mixture of facilities provided may then be seen to be capable of improvement if total value can be increased or total cost reduced, and an optimum mixture obtained when value is maximised (or cost minimised) with a given set of resources.

As an example of a measure of the total cost of ill-health we may cite the health problem index developed by the U.S. Department of Health Education and Welfare (quoted in Parker, 1967), which has been used to measure the effect of devoting more resources to the treatment of particular categories of disease in the international classification. Of particular interest to our discussion is that two of the arguments of which the index is a linear function, namely number of out-patient visits and number of days for which patients' activities are restricted, are given relative values of 3 and 1 respectively. The index, in other words, may take the same value if during any period of time 1 patient is restored to full activity a day earlier or 3 additional out-patient consultations are fitted in. Packer (1968) has similarly suggested a measure of the ineffectiveness of the health service to a given individual which takes the form of a weighted sum of his time spent in various states of disability, impairment of function and premature death. The weight attaching to each state is a measure of the 'disvalue' of being in the state per unit of time, although no specific numerical values are used for the weights.

As an example of the construction of a maximand we may cite the work of Feldstein (1969) which is designed to indicate the mixture of facilities to be chosen for the control of TB. Here each mixture of facilities (isoniazid treatment, prophylactic vaccination, education to promote self-referral of infectives, mass screening, etc., at varying

[1] These two formulations are equivalent if there exists a one-to-one correspondence *between* facilities and health problems.

levels) results in varying levels of different types of benefit (reduced risk of premature death, reduced impairment of function or disability, etc.). The total value of a mixture of facilities is a weighted sum of all the benefits to which the mixture gives rise, the weights or relative values to be decided in accordance with the preferences of the society or its representatives. The extent to which alternative sets of relative values affect the optimum mixture of facilities to be provided is tested by arbitrarily choosing different weighting systems (e.g. a life saved is of equal value in each of four age groups and no value is attached to reduction in disability or impairment of function nor to reduction in the present value of future income).

A further example of the use of a function which relates the mixture of facilities provided to the value of that mixture, and one which is of direct relevance to the problem of the treatment of hospital in-patients, may be found in Feldstein (1967). In this exercise the total value of hospital in-patient facilities is represented by a modified weighted sum of the numbers of discharges and deaths in all specialties in large, acute, non-teaching hospitals for the year 1960/61. Depending on the relative values ascribed to patients discharged from particular specialties, the implied optimum specialty distribution of patients discharged from the average hospital is shown to vary considerably: (i) if patients are considered to be of equal importance in all specialties, e.g. the implied optimum number of discharges and deaths in ENT and T and O surgery is two and a half times the current average number of discharges for these specialties in large, acute hospitals; (ii) if patients in specialties with a higher mean length of stay in hospital or higher average cost of treatment are assumed to be of more value—the implication is that only half as many patients in those specialties should be treated as were in fact being treated in the average acute hospital in 1960/61.

The important features of attempts such as those described above to treat the problems of choice and scarcity in the health service by evaluating the worth of alternative mixtures of facilities, are (i) that arbitrary assumptions require to be made about the relative values of particular facilities, and (ii) that a specific form has to be assumed for the relationship between the mixture of facilities provided and the value of that mixture.

THE OBJECTIVE FUNCTION OF A REGIONAL BOARD

In order to examine one method of eliciting the relative values attached by decision-makers to treating patients in hospital for various disorders, it is now proposed to give some specific content to the general ideas outlined above. We shall suppose that regional hospital boards or their agents make decisions about the numbers and types of in-patients to treat in a way that is rational and in accordance with their preferences. Regional boards, one might say, are assumed to be monolithic optimisers. We shall further assume that the total value of the in-patient facilities provided by a regional board, depends on the numbers and diagnostic categories of patients treated in a given time period, in a way that may be characterised by the following objective function:

$$U = \prod_{i=1}^{n} X_i^{a_i}$$

where X_i denotes the number of patients treated in diagnostic category i. In other words, since

$$\log U = \sum_{i=1}^{n} a_i \log X_i$$

regional boards successfully aim to maximise the weighted sum of the logarithms of numbers of patients treated in all diagnostic categories. Such a characterisation of the preferences of regional boards is, of course, no less arbitrary than the functional forms described in my first section above. It has the advantage, however, of being simple and fairly easily interpretable. Furthermore, if the weights a_i are constrained to lie between 0 and 1, the form of this objective function is such that it implies that an additional patient treated in a particular diagnostic category is preferred more when few such patients are being treated than when many are.[2] Formally, that is to say,

$$\partial U / \partial X_i > 0$$

and

$$\partial^2 U / \partial X_i^2 < 0$$

Since we are interested in the *relative* value attributed to treating patients in different categories (i.e. the ratio a_i/a_j in general) such a constraint should not affect our results. Finally, it will be assumed that the only constraint inhibiting the behaviour of regional boards

[2] And also, of course, that regional boards prefer *cet. par.* to treat more patients in each diagnostic category than fewer.

is that a certain number of bed-days must be occupied, in formal terms,

$$\sum_{i=1}^{n} M_i X_i = B$$

where B is some fixed number of bed-days, equal to the number actually used, and M_i denotes the mean stay of a patient in the ith diagnostic category. In practice, of course, this is most unlikely to be the only, or even a binding constraint, and it should in any case be more realistically expressed in the form of an inequality, a point to which we shall return later. It may also be noted that the stochastic nature of the problem is being completely ignored: the expected value of length of stay, for example, is being used and the fact that M_i takes different values with varying probability is not taken into account.

We are now in a position to determine the relative value attached to treating patients in particular diagnostic categories, since the value weights a_i will be such that a regional board chooses to treat the numbers and categories of patients that are in fact treated subject to the constraint on total bed-days. Denoting by λ an undetermined multiplier, the augmented function

$$F = U + \lambda \left(B - \sum_{i=1}^{n} M_i X_i \right)$$

will have a stationary value where

$$\partial F / \partial X_i = \partial F / \partial X_j = 0$$

i.e.

$$\frac{\partial F}{\partial X_i} = \frac{a_i}{X_i} F - \lambda M_i = 0$$

$$\frac{\partial F}{\partial X_j} = \frac{a_j}{X_j} F - \lambda M_j = 0$$

whence

$$a_i / a_j = M_i X_i / M_j X_j$$

If the stationary value is a maximum, therefore, the value ascribed to treating a patient in one diagnostic category relative to a patient in another category is given by the ratio of total bed-days used to treat patients in the two diagnostic categories.

Whether the stationary value is a maximum or not has to be decided by inspecting the principal minors of the matrix of second derivatives of U bordered by the corresponding first derivatives of $\lambda(B - \sum_i X_i M_i)$, namely:

$$
\begin{vmatrix}
\dfrac{a_1(a_1-1)F}{X_1^2} & \dfrac{a_1 a_2}{X_1 X_2}F & \cdots & \dfrac{a_1 a_n}{X_1 X_n}F & -\lambda M_1 \\[2ex]
\dfrac{a_2 a_1}{X_2 X_1}F & \dfrac{a_2(a_2-1)F}{X_2^2} & \cdots & \dfrac{a_2 a_n}{X_2 X_n}F & -\lambda M_2 \\[1ex]
\vdots & \vdots & & \vdots & \vdots \\[1ex]
\dfrac{a_n a_1}{X_1 X_n}F & \dfrac{a_n a_2}{X_n X_2}F & \cdots & \dfrac{a_n(a_n-1)F}{X_n^2} & -\lambda M_n \\[2ex]
-\lambda M_1 & -\lambda M_2 & \cdots & -\lambda M_n & 0
\end{vmatrix}
$$

For the stationary value to be a maximum the value of this determinant must be negative if the number of diagnostic categories ($= n$) is odd and positive otherwise. The principal minors obtained by deleting the first row and column, first two rows and columns, first three rows and columns, etc., must have determinants of alternating signs. The minor of order $n-2$, for example, must have the same sign as the above matrix. Hence if n is even, for example, the condition is that

$$
\begin{vmatrix}
\dfrac{a_{n-1}(a_{n-1}-1)}{X_{n-1}^2}F & \dfrac{a_n a_{n-1}}{X_n X_{n-1}}F & -\lambda M_{n-1} \\[2ex]
\dfrac{a_n a_{n-1}}{X_n X_{n-1}}F & \dfrac{a_n(a_n-1)}{X_n^2}F & -\lambda M_n \\[2ex]
-\lambda M_{n-1} & -\lambda M_n & 0
\end{vmatrix} > 0
$$

Providing λ is not complex, the evaluation of this determinant shows that the implied condition reduces to

$$\frac{M_n^2 a_{n-1}(a_{n-1}-1)}{X_{n-1}^2} > \frac{M_{n-1}^2 a_n(a_n-1)}{X_n^2}$$

or equivalently, since both M_i^2 and X_i^2 are necessarily positive,

$$\frac{a_{n-1}(a_{n-1}-1)}{(M_{n-1}X_{n-1})^2} > \frac{a_n(a_n-1)}{(M_nX_n)^2}$$

which by virtue of the constraint $0<a_i<1$ for all i implies that

$$\frac{a_{n-1}(a_{n-1}-1)}{a_n(a_n-1)} < \frac{(M_{n-1}X_{n-1})^2}{M_nX_n}$$

Since the first-order condition for a stationary value of F led us to the results that

$$\frac{a_{n-1}}{a_n} = \frac{M_{n-1}X_{n-1}}{M_nX_n}$$

this implies that

$$\frac{a_{n-1}-1}{a_n-1} < \frac{M_{n-1}X_{n-1}}{M_nX_n}$$

in a similar manner the principal minors of higher order may be inspected to derive the implied conditions in terms of the higher powers of bed-days used in particular specialties (i.e. in terms of $(M_iX_i)^n$).

The evaluation of determinants in the manner used above becomes of course a prohibitive task when their order exceeds 3 or 4, but presumably if it were felt worthwhile to derive the further conditions on the coefficients a_i which are implied by the maximisation of F, a computable algorithm could be developed for the purpose. Since the number of diagnostic categories on which information is given in the Hospital In-Patient Enquiry extends to 120, the programming effort involved would clearly be considerable if interest was not to be confined to only a few coefficients and the majority of diagnostic categories 'collapsed' to leave the matrix of second derivatives of relatively low order.

It may also be noted that the preferences of regional boards might be characterised by an objective function of an alternative form or one having arguments other than the numbers of patients treated in each diagnostic category. One might, for example, make use of the quadratic form proposed by Theil (1964):

$$U = \sum_{i=1}^{n} a_i X_i + \tfrac{1}{2}\left(\sum_{i=1}^{n} a_i X_i \right)^2$$

where a_i are value coefficients, X_i numbers treated in diagnostic category i, and a similar constraint as before exists on total bed-days to be used. Similarly one might incorporate length of stay into the objective function on the grounds that for the range of values currently taken by mean length of stay, hospital planners would prefer a lower to a higher value and one might therefore expect U to be a decreasing function of M_i. Clearly, however, the incorporation of further arguments in the objective function (e.g. severity of disorder for which patients are treated) must be matched by their inclusion among the constraints if the implied value weights attaching to these arguments are to be found.

As an example of the sort of inferences that may be drawn about the relative value ascribed to the treatment of various categories of in-patient, we might refer to Hospital In-Patient Enquiry, 1965. Assuming that the condition for a stationary value of F does in fact give us a maximum point, then the relative value of treating a patient in category i is given by

$$\frac{a_i}{a_j} = \frac{M_i X_i}{M_j X_j}$$

which is the ratio of bed-days used for patients in i to those used for patients in j. In the Oxford Region, for instance, the number of bed-days used in 1965 for male patients with varicose veins and hernia and females with cervitis (including erosion) were respectively 335, 1,875 and 311. It follows from our assumptions that relative to the treatment of males with varicose veins, the treatment of male patients for hernia ($a_i/a_k = 5 \cdot 60$) was valued rather more highly than that of female patients for cervitis ($a_j/a_k = 0 \cdot 93$). Furthermore, if the preferences of all regional boards may be characterised by an objective function of identical form, comparisons may be made between regions. The comparable figures to those given above for Oxford were in the Leeds Region 965, 5,650 and 1,159 respectively in 1965, giving relative values of $a_i/a_k = 5 \cdot 86$ and $a_j/a_k = 1 \cdot 20$ (using males treated for varicose veins as numeraire). In the Leeds Region, therefore, the treatment of males for hernia has a relative value considerably higher than the treatment of females for cervitis, but the differential is not so pronounced as that observed in the Oxford Region.

Such illustrations also serve to reveal further difficulties, notably those arising out of the data used. The Hospital In-Patient Enquiry data used above are derived from a 10% sample of all discharges and deaths, so that the number of bed-days used in a particular category and consequently the relative values a_i/a_j are estimates subject to sampling variability. The proportion of total discharges and deaths in each diagnostic category formed by deaths alone may well, of course, vary from one category to another, as may the proportion of patients successfully treated. The value weights derived will therefore by no means be a 'pure' reflection of decision-makers' preferences and the prevalence of disorders, since relative value is unlikely to be independent of the probability of successful treatment.

THE INVERSE-PROGRAMMING APPROACH

It was observed in the preceding section that the constraint on total bed-days available for use, which was there expressed in the form of an equality constraint, could with greater realism be expressed as an inequality, viz.

$$\sum_{i=1}^{n} m_i X_i \leqslant B$$

Furthermore, constraints other than that on bed-days are frequently observed to inhibit the activity of hospitals, groups or regional boards: shortages of nurses and medical staff spring readily to mind as examples. The present section attempts to take account of these features of the situation by regarding hospital authorities as aiming to maximise some objective function subject to maximum available levels of beds, doctors and nurses. The last two constraints may be expressed in the form:

$$\sum_{i=1}^{n} S_i X_i \leqslant S$$

and

$$\sum_{i=1}^{n} t_i X_i \leqslant T$$

respectively, where S_i represents the amount of doctors' time necessary on average for the in-patient treatment of a patient in diagnostic category i, t_i represents the necessary nurses' time for the treatment of such a patient, and S and T are respectively total available doctors' and nurses' time for one year.

By way of illustration it is proposed to construct an example similar to the one used by Feldstein (1967, p. 170). Suppose we have a 16-bed ward which may be used for the in-patient treatment of 2 categories of patient and which is staffed by 2 doctors and 5 nurses. The available resources in bed-days, doctor-sessions and nurse-hours for 1 whole year will then appear something like: bed-days, 5,840; doctor-sessions, 600; and nurse-hours, 10,000. Suppose also that the amounts of each resource necessary on average to complete the treatment of a patient in the two categories (i.e. the technological coefficients) are as follows:

	Bed-Days	Doctor-Sessions	Nurse-Hours
Category 1	16	1	25
Category 2	8	1·5	20

Then our three constraints will take the form:

$$16X_1 + 8X_2 \leqslant 5,840$$

$$X_1 + 1{\cdot}5X_2 \leqslant 600$$

and

$$25X_1 + 20X_2 \leqslant 10,000$$

and the numbers of patients that may be treated in each of the two categories (i.e. the values taken by X_1 and X_2) may be represented by a point in the area bounded by the polygon OABCD in Figure 1 (the integral-valued co-ordinates of points on the boundary ABCD represent the maximum numbers of patients treatable in one year).

Suppose now that the value of the mixture of patients treated in one year may be represented by a weighted sum of the number of patients treated in each category, i.e. the objective function is linear in the relevant range, and the weights denote the relative values ascribed to treating patients in the two categories, viz:

$$U = a_1X_1 + a_2X_2$$

What may be said about the values a_1 and a_2 implicitly used by decision-makers from a knowledge of the distribution of discharges and deaths between the two categories of patient in a particular year?

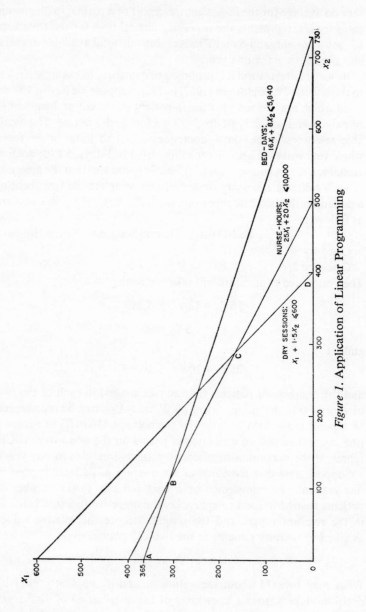

Figure 1. Application of Linear Programming

What, in other words, may be said about the slope of the line between the X_1 and X_2 axes, each of the points on which represents the same value? Assuming that the numbers of patients requiring treatment are large relative to the maxima permitted in view of the constrained resources, and that decision-makers are behaving so as to maximise the total value arising from the treatment of patients in the ward during the year, the number of patients in each category actually treated will be the co-ordinates of some point on the boundary ABCD. If the point lies on one of the sides of the boundary, the objective function will have the same slope as the constraint line of which that side is a section. For example, referring to Figure 1, if the number of patients treated, X_1, was between approximately 310 and 365 and the number X_2 correspondingly somewhere below about 110, the point would lie on the section AB (but not at either A or B) and the objective function would be parallel to the line representing the limited number of bed-days. The values of a_1 and a_2 would therefore be proportional to the technological coefficients representing the number of bed-days required to treat a patient in each category, 16 and 8 respectively in the example used above. Decision-makers, that is to say, may be said in this case to have placed twice as much value on treating patients in the first as on treating those in the second category.

If the number of patients actually treated during the year are the co-ordinates of one of the vertices, A, B, C or D, it will not be possible to place a particular value on the ratio a_1/a_2, but only to set bounds within which it lies. If $X_1 = 160$, $X_2 = 290$ approximately, for example; the point corresponding to these co-ordinates is at C on the diagram. This implies that a_1/a_2 lies between $1/1\cdot5$ and $25/20$, these being the ratios of technological coefficients for doctor-sessions and nurse-hours respectively. In this particular case, of course, we would have learnt very little, since $2/3 \leqslant a_1/a_2 \leqslant 5/4$ and it is not clear which category of patient is reckoned to be of greater importance, or whether both categories are considered to be of equal value ($a_1/a_2 = 1$). Similarly, if the numbers of patients actually treated in the two categories fall at point B ($X_1 = 310$, $X_2 = 110$ approximately) it may be inferred that $25/20 \leqslant a_1/a_2 \leqslant 16/8$, i.e. the value of treating a patient in the first category is considered to be anything from $1\frac{1}{4}$ to 2 times that of treating a patient in the second. If no patient in a particular category is treated (i.e. at A where $X_2 = 0$, or D where $X_1 = 0$) then only the value of the lower bound of the appropriate ratio may be inferred. At point A, for example, only patients in the first category are treated and the ratio a_1/a_2 may take any value not less than $16/8 = 2$.

The example used here, of course, is a trivially simple one involving only two categories of patient and bearing only on the static situation where current behaviour does not affect future values. In principle, however, the method may be generalised to any number of diagnostic categories (n) each constraint defining a hyperplane and the analogue of the boundary ABCD being a hyperpolyhedron in n-dimensional space: assuming decision-makers to behave optimally, the actual distribution of patients among diagnostic categories may be represented by a point on the face of a particular n-dimensional surface (giving unique values a_i/a_j) or by a vertex of a hyperpolyhedron (giving bounds within which a_i/a_j lies). Hawgood (1968), in an interesting application to the relative importance placed on current and future benefits by library planners, also shows how dynamic considerations may be taken into account. A modified simplex algorithm could presumably be used to elicit the relative values by electronic computer, the size of the matrix of technological coefficients and therefore the number of constraints and diagnostic categories being limited only by the computer's capacity.

All this assumes, of course, that data on technological coefficients are readily available, which is manifestly not true. One possible line of approach to the problem of data is to build up a picture from pieces of information to be found in a number of disparate sources. The Platt Report of 1961, for instance (p. 19) has a rough estimate of the number of in-patients that, in conjunction with associated out-patient and emergency work, could be dealt with by a firm of five (two consultants, one registrar and two house officers) working in the average general surgery department of an acute hospital. Similarly, the report by H. A. Goddard published by the Leeds Regional Hospital Board indicates (pp. 32 and 46) that in acute surgical wards in two particular hospitals the total amount of nursing time per bed-day varied from about 140 to 160 minutes. Such data, however, relate to such coarse, heterogeneous specialty groups as general surgery and general medicine. Moreover, any attempt to use them in order to estimate the amounts of various resources necessary for the complete treatment of in-patients requires further information about the relationship between the distribution of duration of stay in hospital and the values taken by these technological coefficients.

It is possible that in the future some of the data required (e.g. on doctor-sessions and operating-theatre time) will become available with the widespread adoption of hospital activity analysis. The method suggested by Feldstein (1967, pp. 171–5), and used by him to estimate the technology matrix (expressed in bed-days and money) for nine broad specialty groups, might in the meantime be applied in conjunction with Hospital In-Patient Enquiry data to derive estimates of the coefficients for each diagnostic category. Briefly, this consists of estimating the coefficients S_i by the linear regression of each resource used on in-patients treated in a particular diagnostic category or specialty:

$$S_h = \sum_{i=1}^{n} S_i X_{ih}$$

for the regression of doctors' sessions in hospital or region h, on patients in category i treated in hospital or region h, for example. The coefficients S_i are then estimated by performing the regression using data relating to a number of hospitals or regions, and similarly for the estimation of coefficients for nurses and other inputs. Although the example used above was cast in terms of a particular ward, there is no reason why such larger units as hospital management committee groups or whole regions should not form the basis.

Finally, a number of difficulties associated with the inverse-programming approach may be mentioned. Hitherto it has been assumed that such inputs as doctor-sessions and nurse-hours are homogeneous and the treatment has been deterministic in the sense that technological coefficients have been assumed to be constant. It would be far more realistic, however, to regard these coefficients as having probability distributions, their value varying both between individual input units (e.g. doctors) and between patients in a given diagnostic category. In principle, the problem can be formulated with stochastic technological coefficients, but the difficulties involved in determining the relative value-weights at which the objective function is maximised become much more severe and frequently prohibitive (see, for example, G. Hadley, 1964, Ch. 5). Similar difficulties arise when the programming problem is non-linear due to the form of the objective function or the stochastic nature of its arguments (e.g. varying incidence as well as patients treated).

FURTHER POSSIBILITIES

In conclusion, mention might briefly be made of further methods by which relative values might be elicited. If the treatment of in-patients is regarded as a process which may be realised in a large number of different possible ways, a sample of 'quasi-observations' of these possible outcomes might be generated by computer simulation. The relative values may then be inferred from these artificial realisations of the process. Where the development of a realistic model of the process results in intractable mathematical problems, indeed, such an approach may be the only possible one.

More directly, one might treat the problem of relative values by a decision-theoretic approach as described in Fishburn (1964). Since questions concerning the relative value attaching to the treatment of particular categories of patient are notoriously 'psychologically oppressive' and difficult to quantify for the individual medical decision-maker, one might couch the question in terms of probability payoffs. For example, if V_{1s} denotes the value of successfully treating a patient of one type, and V_{2s} and V_{2u} respectively the value of successfully and unsuccessfully treating a patient of the second type, one might ask what value of p, the probability of successful treatment for the second type of patient, is such that the condition

$$V_{1s} \geqslant pV_{2s} + (1-p)V_{2u}$$

is just fulfilled. 'Just fulfilled' is used in the sense that a change of p in a particular direction would result in the inequality's being reversed. Hence for some other value of the probability of successful treatment of patients of the second type, say p',

$$V_{1s} \leqslant p'V_{2s} + (1-p')V_{2u}$$

Whence

$$p \leqslant \frac{V_{1s} - V_{2u}}{V_{2s} - V_{2u}} \leqslant p'$$

and bounds are obtained for the relative value attached to treating the two types of patient. For this procedure to work it is necessary for the decision-maker to be able to rank the V_{1s} initially, and for p

not to take values of 0 or 1. The chief difficulty, however, would seem to lie in the eliciting of values from such groups of decision-makers as firms or departments in the sense of the 'Cogwheel' Report: unless unanimity existed among the members of a group, some method of weighting to achieve a consensus would have to be devised.

ACKNOWLEDGEMENTS

I am indebted to the Nuffield Provincial Hospitals Trust for financial support, to Professor J. Wiseman for originally suggesting the idea behind this paper and to Professor A. Williams for some references useful in its preparation.

REFERENCES

Feldstein, M. S., *Economic Analysis for Health Service Efficiency*, Amsterdam 1967 (North-Holland).
Feldstein, M. S., *Health Sector Planning in Developing Countries*, Harvard Institute of Economic Research Discussion Paper, No. 62, Harvard 1969.
Fishburn, P. C., *Decision and Value Theory*, New York 1964 (Wiley).
Hadley, G., *Non-Linear and Dynamic Programming*, Reading (Mass.) 1964 (Addison-Wesley).
Hawgood, J., *Social Benefit Analysis by Inverse Linear Programming*, Paper presented at the European Conference on Technological Forecasting, Glasgow 1968.
Leeds Regional Hospital Board, *Work Measurement as a Basis for Calculating Nursing Establishments*, Part II (Goddard Report), Harrogate 1963.
Ministry of Health, *First Report of the Joint Working Party on the Organisation of Medical Work in Hospitals* ('Cogwheel' Report), London 1967 (H.M.S.O.).
Ministry of Health and Department of Health for Scotland, *Report of the Joint Working Party on Medical Staffing Structure in the Hospital Service* (Platt Report), London 1961 (H.M.S.O.).
Ministry of Health and General Register Office, *Report on Hospital In-Patient Enquiry for 1965* Part I, London 1968 (H.M.S.O.).
Packer, A. H., 'Applying Cost Effectiveness Concepts to the Community Health System', *Operations Research*, vol. 16, No. 2, 1968.
Parker, R. D., *Some Interesting Problems in Medical Operations Research*, School of Hygiene and Public Health, Baltimore 1967.
Theil, H., *Optimal Decision Rules for Government and Industry*, Amsterdam 1964 (North-Holland).

COMMENT ON 'THE IMPLICIT VALUATION OF FORMS OF HOSPITAL TREATMENT'

R. MORLEY
University of Durham

Mr Lavers' interesting paper presents two alternative methods of pinning down the trade-offs between activities in the health service. These comments suggest that the first method is misleading and the second method is insufficient, but that a combination of the second method with an elementary theorem of welfare economics does get us somewhere.

In the second section of the paper there seems to be a minor confusion between making facilities available and using those facilities to provide care. Under most circumstances there will be diminishing marginal benefit from having extra facilities available. (If the marginal benefit from a particular facility would increase if that facility were expanded, and if the facility is already thought to be worth providing at its present level, then it ought to be expanded at the expense of some other facility which is already at a level where marginal benefits are decreasing.) However, we cannot speak of diminishing marginal benefits from the actual care of patients when this care is defined in terms of cures for specific ailments. To do so could imply that the addition to social welfare from curing Mrs Jones's varicose veins was less than that from curing Mrs Smith's. The benefit function is not analogous to a production function. If each cure is defined as being technically equivalent it is also equivalent in value, according to the ethics of the health service. So the actual care provided does not involve diminishing marginal benefits: three cures of the same type are three times as 'good' as one cure, but the trebling of facilities is three times as 'good' only if the expanded facilities are sure to be used to provide three times the number of cures (ignoring improvements in quality).

In addition to the ethical problems of weighting units of hospital services, there are also the usual problems of technical interdependence. An organisation which is the main provider of certain types of care in a locality will tend to add just those activities which are either substitutes or complements to its old activities. Increased use of antenatal facilities means less call on perinatal facilities: the two are substitutes at the margin. Provision of facilities for surgery is complemented by provision of the services of physiotherapists. As a result, the value of a measurable unit of an activity may not be simply a function of the level of that activity; rather it is likely to be a function of the levels of several other activities as well.

The third section of the paper is concerned with a descriptive technique which avoids the problems of the second section by allowing the appropriate decision-makers to judge both ethical matters and matters of technical interdependence. The aim is to obtain some numerical indicators of the relative values which seem to have been placed on hospital activities in the past, so that the administrators can be asked: 'You seem to us to be valuing activities in roughly this way. Is this correct?'. Provided that the data input is correct, that the administrators have understood the question, and that the answer to it is 'yes', the weights together with the data on technology can then be used for optimisation purposes. Then we can reap the advantages of the great versatility of a linear programming approach, using the resulting model to investigate the effects of many alternative policies.

Under certain restricted circumstances it is helpful to find the range of weights (a_j) for large numbers of activities by the following method. Take the matrix of technological coefficients. Eliminate those columns which refer to activities which are at zero level. Eliminate those rows which refer to constraints which are not binding (in the special case where the observed point lies on a 'side' of the set of production possibilities, then all rows except the one referring to the 'side' are eliminated and the solution is simple). The resulting square matrix can be called $T = [t_{ij}]$. Choose the activity which is most suitable to use as numeraire, so one unit of this activity is valued at unity. Suppose this activity is activity 1. Divide each t_{ij} by t_{i1} to obtain a new square matrix $[t_{ij}/t_{i1}]$. The weights on the objective function, relative to the weight on activity 1, are a_j/a_1. The numerical value of this ratio for each activity j lies within the range

$$\underset{i}{\min} \frac{t_{ij}}{t_{i1}} \leqslant \frac{a_j}{a_1} \leqslant \underset{i}{\max} \frac{t_{ij}}{t_{i1}}$$

This is just a matter of running down each column of the $[t_{ij}/t_{i1}]$ matrix and selecting the largest and smallest values.

Unfortunately there are usually many activities which do not require every resource, so T contains many zeroes, and the above method can provide weights that are somewhere between zero and infinity, which we knew already. One method of obtaining precise numerical values for the relative weights is by using marginal cost data and applying the theorems of welfare economics; an alternative approach uses a particular type of geometric average.[1]

I am grateful to Mr A. M. D. Porter, of the Community Medical Care Research Unit, Edinburgh, for the following interim results of an application of the marginal cost/linear programming approach. In a study of the Sunderland maternity services, Porter found that there were fifteen resources which could be limiting expansion. To these fifteen resource constraints there must, of course, be added a 'babies' constraint. There were ten mutually exclusive activities, abbreviated and defined as follows:

DANC Domiciliary Antenatal care, refers only to the A/N care that is provided for expectant mothers at local health authority clinics. It does not include those visits by midwives and health visitors to mothers' homes, nor does it include A/N care provided at GP surgeries. Measured by the total number of 'A/N visits and attendances at clinics' which was 11,234 in 1968.

HANO Hospital Antenatal care (out-patients), refers only to A/N care provided to expectant mothers at the Sunderland Maternity Hospital out-patients clinic. Measured by the total number of attendances which was 20,902 in 1968.

HANI1 Hospital Antenatal care (in-patients), refers to those ex-
HANI2 pectant mothers who are provided with specialist in-patient
HANI3 care during their A/N stage of pregnancy. Measured by the number of cases discharged from the hospital wards. In 1968, there were 491 such cases, being:

---

[1] See Ch. 3 and Appendix 1, respectively, of John Hawgood and Richard Morley, *Evaluating the Benefits of University Libraries*, Durham 1969.

364 HANI1 with an average length of stay of 6·6 bed-days
43 HANI2 with an average length of stay of 1·6 bed-days
84 HANI3 with an average length of stay of 6·0 bed-days

DCC   Domiciliary Confinement care, refers to the care which a mother receives when she is delivered at home. It also includes any A/N home visits which she may receive from the midwife or health visitor, and the nursing care provided to mother and child for the first ten days post-delivery. It does not include any subsequent care the mother or her child may receive. Measured by the total number of cases delivered at home, 1,330 in 1968.

HEDC   Hospital Early-discharge care, refers to mothers booked for confinement at the Sunderland Maternity Hospital and whose condition allows them to be discharged after only 48 hours. This policy of reduced hospitalised care requires close co-operation with the local health authority who provide nursing care to the mother and baby until the tenth day. Measured by the total number of cases discharged after 48 hours, which was 351 in 1968.

HNSC   Hospital Normal-stay care, refers to those mothers booked for a ten-day stay in hospital, although many are discharged before the ten days are completed. In 1968, 2,313 mothers were discharged from hospital between the third and tenth days, with an average length of stay of 8·0 days.

HLSC   Hospital Long-stay care, refers to cases requiring stays in hospital of more than ten days, 119 in 1968. The range was from eleven to twenty-six days, with an average length of stay of 12·3 days.

HPNI   Hospital Postnatal care (in-patients), refers to the small number of women who have to be admitted to the maternity hospital for specialist post-delivery care. In 1968, there were 21 mothers discharged after such care, with an average length of stay of 8·0 days.

In Table 1, row 1 gives the marginal cost of these activities. On the assumption that the ratio of marginal costs will equal the ratio of shadow prices, these marginal costs can be used as the weights on the objective function. Given the constraints, these weights would predict the level of activities shown in row 2. The predicted provision does

Table 1. Interim Results

	DANC	HANO	HANI1	HANI2	HANI3	DCC	HEDC	HNSC	HLSC	HPNI
1. Marginal costs	0·3	0·3	12·5	11·7	14·4	19·3	18·0	27·2	35·7	18·7
2. Predicted provision	0	20,893	343	0	1,151	1,236	1,434	1,443	0	0
3. Actual provision	11,234	20,902	364	43	84	1,330	351	2,313	119	21
4. Implied weights	0·3	0·3	3·7	9·5	9·5	19·3	14·2	19·6	25·3	12·5
5. Implied weights HEDC = 1	0·02	0·02	0·3	0·7	0·7	1·4	1·0	1·4	1·8	0·9

not correspond well with the actual provision as shown in row 3. The model is sensitive to changes in some of the weights, but other weights require fairly large changes to result in changed activity levels (the MPS print-out gives useful hints on sensitivity).

There are several possible reasons for this lack of correspondence between rows 2 and 3. The time period over which the marginal costs are calculated may differ from that taken into account intuitively by the decision-makers. Also, the decision-makers of a social institution may be taking externalities into account. And, of course, the decisions may not be optimal.

Row 4 of the table shows the weights which will lead to a linear programming solution which corresponds to the actual observed level of provision. As shown above, there will be a range of weights which will predict any given blend of levels of provision. The weights in this row are those which are nearest to the marginal costs but which will still yield the observed levels as a solution.

Row 5 is in the same ratio as row 4, but with a convenient activity treated as numeraire, in this case the 48-hour stay in Hospital (HEDC). So row 5 gives the trade-offs between activities in an easily discussable form. To take one example, this could lead to a constructive debate on why home confinements (DCC) should be 'valued' more highly than the 48-hour stay in hospital, contrary to national policy and the opinions of specialist obstetricians.

INCREASING THE EFFICIENCY OF IN-PATIENT TREATMENT

M. A. HEASMAN

Research and Intelligence Unit, Scottish Home and Health Department

INTRODUCTION

There are very wide variations in the approach that different consultants have to the stay in hospital of their patients in this country today. Figures 1, 2 and 3 provide evidence for this in Scotland for a single disease, 'hernia'. Data for other diseases show variations which are just as wide. These data refer only to male patients treated for hernia in surgical units. Each dot in these figures represents one consultant who has had at least twenty patients with inguinal hernia under his care during 1967. All consultants shown work principally in acute hospitals of more than 100 beds. Figure 1 shows the percentage of patients with a diagnosis of inguinal hernia who had an operation during their stay in hospital. It is obvious that a few patients will be found on admission to be unfit for operation, but the variation here is so wide that there is a strong case for believing that in at least some cases the patient had been inadequately assessed prior to admission and that hospital resources had been wasted thereby. Figures 2 and 3 present different aspects of the same question. The former deals with the proportion of patients who were admitted three days or more before operation. Again it shows a very wide variation and again one is bound to ask the question: why were a relatively large number of consultants admitting a considerable proportion of their patients such a long time prior to surgery? In some cases, and certainly for some diseases, prolonged preparation may be desirable, but this should be relatively rare for hernia. Is there any advantage in a long pre-operative stay for the remainder? Prima facie the answer is no, and if this is borne out by detailed clinical study this would seem to reveal an unnecessary waste of clinical resources. Using duration of stay after operation, Figure 3 shows another large scatter for different consultants. Some consul-

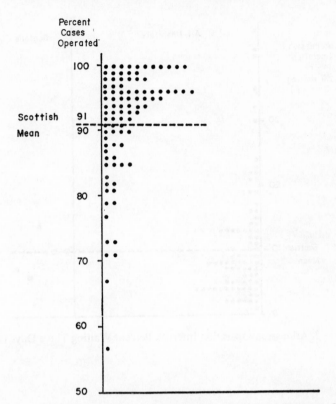

Figure 1. General Surgery. Operation-Hernia-Males. Percent Cases Operated

tants discharge their patients after three days and others keep them for twelve days (other consultants operate on selected patients with simple hernias in out-patient departments, and these data are not included). These three figures and generalisation from them raise important medical and economic questions, which the remainder of this paper will discuss.

It is possible that a longer (or a shorter) stay might have beneficial effects on the patient, as measured by date of return to work, recurrence rate, post-operative complication rates, etc. In general, these effects can best be measured by controlled clinical trials, in which patients are allocated at random to different treatment groups and followed up for as long a period as necessary. An example of such a

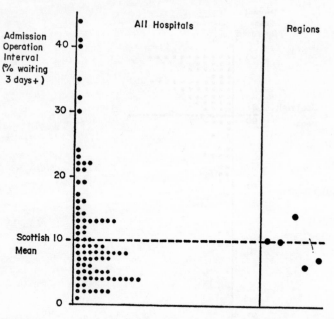

Figure 2. Admission-Operation Interval. Percent Waiting Three Days Plus

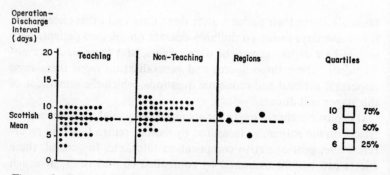

Figure 3. General Surgery. Operation-Hernioplasty-Males. Operation-Discharge Interval in Days

study is that by Morris, Ward and Handyside.[1] Such clinical trials are time-consuming although necessary procedures.

Peculiar local conditions, such as an outbreak of cross-infection, may have resulted in an apparently abnormal practice which is easily explainable in the light of local knowledge. Similar discrepancies may result from problems of local administration. For this reason the Scottish Home and Health Department is particularly careful, when pointing out variations of this sort, not to introduce any note of criticism of individual consultants. Data on the individual consultant are sent to him in confidence and it is hoped that he will compare his own data with that of his colleagues or with that of a regional or national norm. It is hoped that such intra-professional discussions and the implications of group responsibility that they carry, will in the long run result in a general increase in efficiency through improvement in the utilisation of resources.

At the same time as these medical implications are being considered it is important that some consideration be given to the economic implications of variations in consultant performance. The discussion on this point will be divided into two parts: (i) the need for data and its possible uses, and (ii) the economic means by which changes in performance might be encouraged.

THE NEED FOR DATA

Using the current hospital costing data it can be calculated that with a national average stay in hospital (for male patients) of ten days for hernia, the total cost of the hospital stay in Scotland would be £399,260 (at the costs obtaining in large, acute, non-teaching hospitals). If on the other hand the average stay could be reduced to the lower quartile (eight days) the total cost would be £319,408, a saving of £80,000 (Morris *et al.* were comparing six-day and one-day stays). With present resources this saving would immediately be redeployed in other ways. It should be pointed out however that the hospital cost is but a proportion of the total cost of the disease to the nation. In 1967 there were 283,660 days lost through sickness due to hernia in working males in Scotland. At current rates this costs something over £250,000 per year (assuming 80% of men of working age are married) in social security benefits. In Great Britain, 3 million days are lost and costs are of the order of £2½ million. In addition

[1] *Lancet*, vol. 1, p. 681, 1968.

there are further unknown costs of domiciliary treatment and the cost involved in lost production.

Data which exist at the moment only permit calculation of the effect of differences in consultant performance insofar as hospital costs are concerned. The effect of shortening hospital stay could, however, have important effects on total sickness costs for a disease. Only detailed investigation will reveal whether a shorter stay in hospital results in an earlier or a delayed return to work. It is important to know this. Intuitively, however, it seems likely that the effect will be small in either direction. Nevertheless intuition is not a substitute for measurement. What seems more likely to be affected by a shortened duration of stay is the waiting time prior to admission.

If the average duration of stay of surgical patients could be reduced by a relatively small amount then, in theory, and provided the appropriate resources are not overstretched thereby, the waiting-list for admission to surgical beds would very soon be cleared. Unfortunately there appears to be a difference between theory and practice here, for just as Logan's 'third law of thermodynamics' states that a hospital bed must be kept warm, so there are some dimly understood factors which seem to ensure that in the United Kingdom a waiting-list remains of approximately constant size. Leaving aside the question of danger and discomfort caused by delay in treatment, at the moment there are no data available on the working time lost by patients on a hospital waiting-list. Such data could be made available by the linkage of hospital statistics to social security statistics. The data that would be made available thereby would considerably facilitate economic studies in medical care. It is to be hoped that the day is not far distant when this might be possible.

Once the economic effects of different treatment regimes (including length of stay) can be assessed relatively easily then together with knowledge of the medical effects it will become easier to assess an optimum regime using cost-benefit techniques. It may be that we shall have to await the results of such studies before professional pressures will build up to such an extent that there is any rapid improvement in the use of resources, if indeed such improvement is possible. Is there anything that can be done then?

THE QUESTION OF INCENTIVES
It is important to distinguish efficiency and effectiveness in this con-

text. By efficiency is meant the reduction in the cost per case treated. This can include total costs, however defined, and may also be limited to hospital treatment or may include domiciliary treatment as well. Effectiveness, on the other hand, relates to the outcome of treatment whether this is measured by survival, restoration of function, relief of pain, etc.

It must be made quite clear that, with extremely rare exceptions, improvements in efficiency of treatment cannot be achieved by administrative fiat. They must result from professional acceptance of the desirability for change. Pressures from group discussion are the most widely accepted method, but economic pressures might have a place.

The health service, as at present functioning, apparently has built into it disincentives to increased efficiency of medical care. For the same output an inefficient hospital or ward uses up more resources than an efficient one, and the latter by its very efficiency tends to release resources which become available for reallocation and may be used to prop up the crumbling edifice of the former. The system of block allocations is almost bound to result in this. What is needed is a device whereby an efficient team has an incentive to do better. It is usually suggested that incentives in the form of 'bonus payments' to increase personal salaries are completely excluded and that incentives should be in the form of extra money made available for the purchase of equipment or, say, extra secretarial staff.

This is not an easy problem, but it is one that is worth study. It would seem that divisional budgets alone are not the answer, because one of the paradoxes of health service care is that increased efficiency almost inevitably leads to increased annual costs. The cost per patient will fall but the cost per patient-day will probably rise because the patient is, on the average, in need of more intensive care during his stay in hospital. An increase in throughput therefore is likely to increase annual costs.

If this is so then increase in efficiency and any reward for this will depend for its introduction upon an acceptable measurement of the former. Such a measure must, of course, be acceptable both to the medical profession and to their nursing colleagues, and it may be that combined medical and nursing teams would be the most acceptable organisational device in order to distribute benefit from any such schemes.

It is probably not impossible to assess efficiency in in-patient medical care; presumably this will depend upon various measures of increased throughput in relation to the staff and beds available. Where the problem will arise is in the conflict between efficiency and effectiveness. This might appear to be paradoxical, but a little thought will show that it is not so. All will agree that a unit with a high throughput but a low 'cure' rate would be a dangerous unit. Even under ideal conditions there must come a point where greater efficiency will lead to lower effectiveness. What we do not know is the shape of the efficiency/effectiveness relationship. Three possibilities are given in Figure 4, but these are purely hypothetical. Presumably each

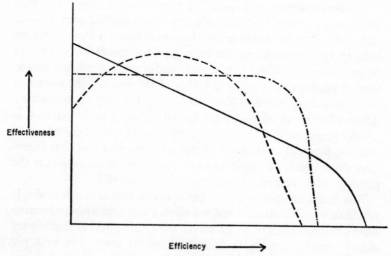

Figure 4. Possible Efficiency/Effectiveness Curves for Hospital In-Patient Treatment

efficiency/effectiveness curve would have to be built up on a disease-specific basis, with varying criteria for effectiveness being used. For example, one can visualise effectiveness measurements for treatment of hernia being developed from an amalgam of: speed of return to full activity, recurrence rate and (rarely) mortality; such a measurement would have to take into account the age, general condition and occupation of the patient. On the other hand, the effectiveness of palliative treatment for cancer would presumably be derived from the length of time and the extent by which troublesome symptoms have been relieved. It is obvious therefore that measurement of effectiveness is very largely a medical problem, although the patient and the social pressures that are created by public opinion may also play their part. The measurement of efficiency is still largely medical, if only because of the relationship between the two. However the economist has an important role to play in costing both efficiency and effectiveness and in questioning some of the implicit medical assumptions.

From a medical viewpoint, therefore, the problem of variation in consultant performance (or hospital activity) is one which requires better basic data, but also data which are linked with events occurring outside the hospital. With these data, efforts can then be made to introduce a more realistic appraisal of the total costs of various treatment regimes. Further, they may be of value in the examination of 'incentive bonus' schemes in medical work, difficult though they may be to introduce. The difficulty appears to lie not in obtaining agreement on measures of efficiency, but on their relationship to measures of effectiveness.

THE COSTING OF HOSPITAL VERSUS DOMICILIARY TREATMENT

Although this paper so far has been developed from a single point, that of variations in consultant performance, it is not difficult to extend the argument further. It is particularly difficult to assess the value of hospital stay with chronic invalids, especially in the mentally subnormal, geriatric and psycho-geriatric field. The decision to hospitalise a particular individual appears to rest primarily on a combination of medical and 'moral' grounds. While there is some dispute over the medical grounds, the moral grounds are the ones over which there is the most argument, the role of relatives and the provision of community support being paramount in the discussion. It would seem that this will long remain the case, but economists may have something to offer in this field.

It must be assumed that on a cost-benefit basis a very large proportion of chronic care can expect to show no return. Presumably this is covered in theory by the insurance principle. But there have been no studies of the total cost of illness of individual patients who are chronically sick. In theory, with sufficient support, no chronically ill patient need ever be in hospital, unless he does require specialised equipment available only there, nor need relatives be at all incommoded. In practice, however, it is obvious that there must come a point at which it is no longer economic for an individual to be kept in the community. The problem is to define approximately where that point falls. It is probable that this could be done if the medical profession were able to devise a scale of mental and physical function, allied to the support needed for each point on the scale (the Government Social Survey's current disability study may be a good point from which to start) and if economists were able to cost the support needed. The problem lies not in the measurement of the cost of a visit by, for example, a district nurse, but in transfer into meaningful and presumably money terms of the strain on relatives and neighbours and all that this implies.

Various alternative methods of providing services need to be studied with no preconceived notions as to their applicability, varying from visits by domiciliary, medical nursing and social workers, through day (or night) hospitals, residential local authority care, right up to care in hospital which approaches that given in intensive nursing care. Any studies of this sort must be related to individual patients if only because the transfer of a group of patients, say from geriatric hospital to residential care, will inevitably increase the average cost of those remaining.

This paper has concentrated basically on one point, the cost of in-patient care, and has suggested the need, in this respect, to study the total cost of sickness. Without these extra data (mostly obtainable through linkage techniques) any attempt to improve hospital efficiency will probably be unacceptable. Nevertheless there are problems in efficiency/effectiveness relationships, 'incentive bonus' schemes and cost-effectiveness of domiciliary and hospital care, which require economic expertise and help.

COMMENT ON 'INCREASING THE EFFICIENCY OF IN-PATIENT TREATMENT'

R. J. MILNE
University of Glasgow

The main emphasis of Mr Heasman's stimulating paper is on incentives and the scope for their implementation of policy, but before the question of incentives is discussed I wish to make three comments on the rest of the paper:

(1) In his assessment of costs Mr Heasman has made two errors. He has mistaken transfer payments, in this case social security, for real costs, i.e. the use of resources. Social security systems certainly require resources to be used, but this is not to say that payments are part of the resources. If he had meant to measure the loss of earnings by using social security expenditure, then it is mistaken also to include the loss of production. These are different ways of representing loss of output, and only one should be included.

(2) With reference to the 'savings' of hospital costs from reducing the average duration of stay, the savings implied indicates a situation where the hospital resources which have been freed are no longer employed. This situation may only exist after a considerable period of time. The more immediate consequence of reducing the average duration of stay may be to increase the rate of admissions—the savings implied here are the greater benefits—and increase the use of resources. This latter point is made later in the paper.

(3) Some concern was expressed about the validity of cost-benefit techniques in deciding between hospital and domiciliary care of chronic invalids. Without wishing to ignore the considerable difficulties of such estimations, it seems to me that the basis for such a comparison must lie on the assumption that the quality of provision is the same at home or in the hospital. The quality of provision refers not only to the invalid, but also to the relatives and neighbours, who are at risk for stress.

221

The main emphasis of Mr Heasman's paper has been upon incentives and the conflict between 'efficiency' and 'effectiveness'. The terms 'efficiency' and 'effectiveness' are not commonly used by economists, but we will follow his definitions. The conflict between efficiency and effectiveness arises when increased efficiency can only be achieved by decreasing the effectiveness of treatment, i.e. there must be a trade-off between efficiency and effectiveness. Whether the conflict is real or imaginary does not affect the appropriateness of using incentives, although the choice of incentives may be affected. However, there will certainly be different implications for public policy.

We now indicate the scope for reducing duration of stay, one measure of efficiency suggested by Mr Heasman, who has shown that duration varies widely. Whether such a degree of variation is regarded as desirable or not, such variation implies that duration is subject to important influences. Three influences, two of which have an empirical basis, are here indicated:

(1) In Britain the decision on length of stay in hospital is largely determined by the consultant, although the patient may still discharge himself. This assumption is held by Mr Heasman and is consistent with the information given in his Figures 1, 2 and 3. Research could undoubtedly find that there was a systematic explanation for some of the variation in the physician's decision, and that some of the influences were subject to government control. Without wishing to anticipate the true explanations, economic incentives might be considered. No direct incentives exist yet to encourage consultants to reduce duration of stay, although there may be indirect influences such as whether the consultant's appointment is full- or part-time.

(2) As mentioned, the patient has discretion to discharge himself. Experience in the U.S.A., where a large part of the financial burden is borne by the patient, suggests patients are sensitive to the cost of hospital care. In Figure 1 we show the distribution of cases, for a given condition, in public and private hospitals by duration of stay. There is a marked difference in the two distributions. The distribution for the public hospital is unimodal, rising and falling evenly from the peak. In contrast, although the distribution for the private hospital is also unimodal, it falls sharply from the peak after, say, twenty-one day's stay in hospital. The singular behaviour of the distribution for the private hospitals can be explained by the fact that

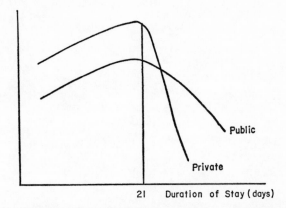

Source: Dr F. Boddy, Department of Social Medicine, University of Glasgow.
Figure 1. Distribution of Cases by Duration of Stay in Public and Private Hospitals

hospital insurance coverage for this condition only lasts for twenty-one days.

(3) There is evidence to suggest that the number of cases treated is directly related to the quantity and quality of medical care provided.[1] Surprisingly, the same study did not find that the variation in the provision of nursing care was insufficient to make any impact on the number of cases treated.[2] If one can assume that the bed size of the ward or hospital is given, as this study did, then the number of cases treated is inversely related to the duration of stay. Thus it has been demonstrated that greater medical provision can reduce duration of stay.

We have attempted to indicate that duration of stay in hospital is sensitive to factors within the control of public policy. However, there is scope for much more research to identify other factors. Any implications require the important qualification: that the reduction of duration of stay is only part of a responsible policy. Effective implementation by, say, charging patients after a given period in hospital, may put unreasonable burdens on those whom we wish to help most.

[1] M. S. Feldstein, *Economic Analysis for Health Service Efficiency*, Amsterdam 1967, p. 98 (North-Holland).
[2] *Ibid.*

Chapter V

SOCIAL ACCOUNTING AND OPERATIONAL RESEARCH IN MEDICAL CARE

H

ECONOMICS AND OPERATIONAL RESEARCH IN THE HEALTH SERVICES

R. N. CURNOW

Head, Department of Applied Statistics and Director, Nuffield Operational Research (Health Services) Unit, University of Reading

INTRODUCTION

In this paper I shall refer, although only in the most general terms, to the work of the Nuffield Operational Research (Health Services) Unit at Reading University. As this is not the place to comment in detail on specific projects, I wish to pick out and attempt to categorise those aspects of the work done by us and others in the same field, that have, or should have, an economic content. Also, I shall ask what contributions economists can make to the solution of some of the problems that arise. Many of the problems are at a rather low or local level of organisation but presumably this does not preclude them from the attention of economists. Much of my material could be described as being within the definition of cost-benefit analysis.

THE COST OF FACILITIES

The earliest applications of operational research techniques to health service problems were concerned with appointment systems in out-patients clinics and in GP waiting-rooms. The decisions required involved financial considerations only insofar as it was necessary to strike a balance between the time spent by patients waiting to see a consultant or a GP and the time of the doctor that might be wasted if there were no patients waiting to be seen. Other examples of applications of operational research where the available resources are fixed and therefore there are few financial considerations, are problems concerned with the more efficient use of existing facilities. These facilities may be wards, beds, X-ray machines or operating theatres. Clearly there is no balancing of financial advantages and disadvantages here. The resources should be used as efficiently as possible.

Other applications of operational research techniques in hospitals have been concerned with the calculation of the number of beds required to meet variable demands such as arise in intensive care units, accident and emergency wards and maternity units. Here there clearly is an economic balance to be struck. The costs of providing extra beds need to be balanced against the costs and other less easily quantified disadvantages of having to find additional beds at times of peak demand. In intensive care units, the extra bed or beds may not be in the unit itself and therefore the care provided may be of reduced quality. How do we decide between the costs of extra beds and the disadvantages of providing hurried or less satisfactory care? The use of relatively arbitrary standards, e.g. that the number of beds must meet their demand 95% of the time, can disguise rather than illuminate the real problems of balance and compromise. These examples all concern the provision of care that must be provided at some level or other. There is no question of deciding to provide no care—the question is the level of care. What is the medical effect of a lowered level of care and how can it be measured on the same scale as financial costs? Similar considerations apply when we consider decisions that have to be made about the provision of facilities that are not absolutely essential but are obviously advantageous. How do we balance the cost of extra X-ray machines against the consequent reduction of time in being examined and in time waiting in X-ray departments? How do we balance the cost of the extra equipment against the advantages to patients of, for example, increased testing facilities in pathology laboratories, extra and more sensitive X-ray equipment, more maternity beds in hospitals and GP units or additional operating theatres? More pointedly, how do we decide the optimum level of investment in operational research?

To take extra facilities for biochemical tests as an example of this category of problem, can we quantify their advantages in terms of improved diagnosis and treatment and in terms of shorter lengths of stay in hospital? Can we quantify the contributions that these extra facilities may well make in the future to our knowledge about the origins, progression and treatment of disease? I am concerned that insufficient thought and investment may be given to recording and analysing the relevance and use made of results of new testing facilities. A similar type of problem arises again in considering the appropriate average length of stay required for different types of patient. Can we compare on the same scale the increased number of patients that can be given treatment for a fixed total number of beds and staff available, against the possible disadvantages of returning some patients home too soon? Can we estimate the costs of providing sufficient care at the patients home, via the GP and the community health services, to justify the earlier discharge home? The early discharge of mothers and babies home after a hospital confinement is an obvious example of this kind of problem. The whole concept of progressive care also involves similar considerations. The decreased costs must be set against the possible disadvantages to the patients of early transfer from expensive acute beds to pre-discharge or convalescent beds and then home.

There are very few occasions when alternative methods of providing a particular service involve roughly equal total costs. One example in the work of the Nuffield Unit was in a study of an ambulance service. A considerable variation in the proportion of non-urgent patients carried by the hospital car service resulted in roughly the same total cost of running the ambulance and hospital car services. At the same time it was clear that an increase in the proportion of patients carried by hospital cars would be beneficial to a great number of patients. This may raise other issues about manpower and redundancy that are economic in nature!

NEED VERSUS DEMAND AND PRIORITIES

The importance of distinguishing between the needs of individuals for particular types of medical care and their demand for it is clear. We are convinced that, wherever possible, individual need must be identified and priorities established for the meeting of that need. We are hoping shortly to undertake a study of the needs of all people aged over 65 in a particular area. The plan is that every person over 65 should be visited and assessed not only in terms of the services required by that particular person, but also in terms of the time at which they should be revisited and their needs reassessed. We are hoping to establish a central register of information about this particularly vulnerable section of the community and attach a priority to the meeting of each individual need. This will not only be useful in terms of the planning of future services but will, we hope, result in a better allocation of scarce resources to those people who can benefit most from receiving them. The cost of the scheme would be recovered if, as seems likely, it saved or delayed one or two people from the need for institutional care. We hope that this central register will be a centre of information which will be kept up-to-date by the receipt of information from many sources and will be used to decide on the allocation of additional resources, or resources that are no longer needed by other people, to those who most urgently need them. It is, of course, inevitable that total need will exceed demand and will exceed the resources available to meet the total need. We recognise the great difficulties involved in avoiding the false raising of hopes about the provision of services. Information about unmet need will, of course, be useful in future planning. We consider that there is a considerable case for the increased education of the general public in the necessity for identifying and attaching priorities to individual need and explaining that not all needs can be met with existing resources. One example of studying need rather than demand in our own work was a survey to find out how much 'hidden demand' there was for general surgery in a particular area because GPs were referring their patients outside the area, or privately or not referring them at all on account of the long waiting-lists. We have been able to quantify this hidden demand and this will be useful in the proper planning of the future facilities needed for general surgery in the area. A simple survey of this kind can often be informative.

There has been a considerable amount of interest recently in the selection of patients for observation and treatment. Recent work on medical screening has highlighted some of the economic questions that arise. Again we have 'need versus demand' and the question of priorities. We, like many others, have been studying the way in which expectant mothers are selected for hospital, GP unit and domiciliary confinements in a certain area. We are interested to see to what extent the local 'rules' are being followed. We are also trying to see whether those mothers who are delivered in hospital are in fact those who benefit most from a hospital confinement. We are doing this by gathering information about all the births in the area and studying the incidence of perinatal mortality, the development of complications and, to some extent, the health of the mother and child following delivery. We hope that it will be possible to develop a better method of assessing the priority of each expectant mother for a hospital confinement. Then, if in a particular area the number of expectant mothers likely to have different values of this assessment rating can be estimated, the implications of the provision of a certain number of maternity beds can be related to the level of risk that can be guaranteed a hospital confinement. How can the optimal proportion of hospital confinements be calculated, given its implications for the levels of risk to those mothers who will still have to be delivered at home? If nothing else, this study should, like many others in this field, highlight the real decisions that are and have to be made. One by-product of an operational research study is often the clearer understanding of the purposes of the service concerned and of the criteria by which its performance can be judged.

At present many hospital beds are occupied by elderly patients who have developed conditions that can be contained but not cured. This is preventing the treatment of younger people, some of whom may, as a result, later need hospitalisation and therefore in their turn block acute beds. Can this be expressed in economic terms? Allowing for reduced earnings and dependence on state support would be easy by comparison. Along similar lines, how can the effects of health education and other measures of preventive medicine be quantified?

'WHO DOES WHAT?'

Clearly, many of the most difficult problems in the organisation and administration of the health services arise from questions of the 'Who does what?' variety. Are junior hospital doctors doing work that could be done by nursing staff, are GPs doing work that could be done by community nurses, are ambulances doing work that could be done by hospital cars, are consultants seeing patients in their outpatient clinics that could be seen by a GP, are the mentally subnormal under the care of consultant psychiatrists when they really need supervision by people with different types of skills altogether? Operational research has a contribution to make here in assisting in the classification of the needs of patients so that the medical profession can assess whether the particular level and type of medical attention they are at present receiving are most appropriate and justifiable given the competing demands on the limited total available resources of trained manpower. These questions of 'Who does what?' are somewhat similar to questions already discussed about the use of expensive facilities. What proportion of the mentally subnormal population need expensive hospital facilities? What proportion of patients who occupy acute beds could in fact be treated in pre-discharge wards or even at home? How can we quantify the disadvantages of less skilled attention and less expensive facilities so that these can be compared with their costs?

THE ROLE OF OPERATIONAL RESEARCH

We see the main role of operational research as providing quantitative information about the likely effects of changes in organisation or in facilities. Experimentation in different forms of organisation and in the provision of differing amounts and types of equipment is generally impossible. Mathematical analytical solutions are rarely possible. A detailed study of a present situation followed by statistical analysis, often using simulation techniques, can provide some estimates of the possible effects of change. It is difficult to see how decisions can be made about alternative proposals without that information of this kind is available. It is not for operational research to become involved in questions such as whether a hospital should have a terminal care unit; this question raises many medical, social and ethical questions that are entirely outside the province of the economist or the operational research specialist. What we can do is to provide those who have to make these difficult decisions with information about how many beds would be needed to establish such a unit and what effect this would have on existing wards where terminal care is at present provided.

Sometimes the effects of change can be calculated quite simply, using data already available. However, questions concerned with, for example, the optimal siting of ambulance stations or the effects of new motorways and industrialisation on the ambulance service and accident wards, provide cases where a great deal of thought, data collection and analysis are clearly necessary. They are also good examples of the impossibility of experimentation in deciding questions of this kind. What are the consequences for a patient, in terms of survival and recovery, of delays of given magnitude in being reached by an ambulance? How are these consequences to be measured on the same scale as monetary costs?

We have become increasingly involved over the last year or so with problems arising in the organisation, by local public health authorities and GPs, of the community health services. We are, for example, hoping to study the best way in which available resources, manpower and finance should be deployed and co-ordinated in the community nursing service. We are thinking here particularly of the changes consequent on the attachment of nurses to health centres and general practices. The effects of changes in the organisation of local government services and in local government itself, will have very considerable effects on the health services and these need to be predicted and investigated as a matter of considerable urgency. The development of New Towns provides an ideal opportunity for the establishment of information systems covering hospitals and community services, that can provide the data necessary for testing new ways of organising local health services and also provide a more efficient way to predict, identify and meet individual needs. We are hoping that our scheme to develop a register for the elderly will be taken up by one of the New Towns. It will clearly be much easier to establish such a register in a completely new area.

I have no space to discuss the work of the Nuffield Unit on manpower problems, but we have been studying the implications of the Todd Report for the postgraduate training of doctors. We have been trying to calculate the number of training posts needed to meet the requirements for training. We have done this for all specialties considered together and are now involved in more detailed studies concerned with training posts and career structure in particular specialties. In addition to these detailed studies there is a place, we believe, for simple surveys. We have recently carried out an investigation to discover why staff members of a particular group of hospitals left. This did provide some rather simple and obvious answers but was useful to the hospital administrators in terms of the need to consider improving certain staff facilities and working conditions. It is proving more difficult to put right the complaints about pay and hours!

By far the greatest problem with operational research is to get any conclusions implemented. The lack of hierarchy of authority within hospitals has been a serious problem in bringing pressures to bear to bring about beneficial changes. As already stated, our main purpose is to quantify the likely effects of change, but this information must be seen by colleagues in other departments of the hospital and by hospital administrators so that it can be seen in the overall pattern of the whole hospital. We very much hope that the new structures proposed as part of the 'Cogwheel' report will assist in promoting more rational discussions and, where appropriate, implementation of our recommendations. We are fortunate in Reading in that we have become involved in the 'Cogwheel' committee structure in the local group of hospitals and have had a great deal of co-operation from the hospitals, local GPs and the public health authorities. We hope that there will in future be a greater demand from the Department of Health and the regional boards for properly argued cases about extra staff and the purchase of extra equipment and facilities, including buildings. As in so many fields, financial pressures, though unpopular, can bring about changes that are long overdue.

The two main questions I should like to see discussed by economists, concerning the kind of problems that we have encountered, are:

1. How can we measure and compare the effects of different types of investment in facilities and manpower when the effects are measured on patients and their relatives and are seen primarily in terms of the alleviation of suffering or the postponement of death? You may assume that the medical effects are known although this is rarely true!

2. How can financial pressures be so directed that they result in a more efficient use of available facilities and manpower and a more rational, efficient and effective organisation of the provision, and planning of the future provision, of medical care?

COMMENT ON 'ECONOMICS AND OPERATIONAL RESEARCH IN THE HEALTH SERVICES'

D. K. GRAY

Department of Health and Social Security

The proposition is put forward in Mr Luck's paper on 'Decision-Making Within Hospitals' that the National Health Service is an organism which, because of the pressures created by the persistent gap between demand and supply, has a neurotic tendency to be concerned with survival rather than economic efficiency. Professor Curnow's paper may be interpreted as coming to the same conclusion, albeit he makes a number of other observations as well.

One may agree with Professor Curnow's plea for the need for operational research studies in the health service field; and for the inclusion of economic analysis in these studies. One may also have sympathy for his desire to see more evidence of positive management direction, one consequence of the alleged lack of which appears to be delay in the adoption of recommendations based on operational research studies. Professor Curnow sees a need for more discipline and more incentives.

Since both Professor Curnow's and Mr Luck's papers imply concern at an apparent lack of 'will to economic efficiency' in the NHS organisation, it may be useful to consider this as a specific subject.

However, I think that neither paper was aimed so much at the qualitative aspects of efficiency (what Mr Heasman has called effective treatment) as at the quantitative (cost-effectiveness) aspects. To narrow the field of discussion still further I propose to ignore distinctions between those outputs of service which may be said to have an investment value (GNP outputs) and those which have a consumer value only; in other words, an unsubtle interpretation will be put upon cost-effectiveness.

Collectively, the factors which lead to the diagnosis of managerial neurosis may be summarised in the observation that 'the NHS cannot afford to be efficient'. If it can be shown that there are physical rather than psychological causes for the alleged malady, it may be claimed that the diagnosis is invalid, or at most only partially justified.

There are several 'physical' reasons why optimum cost-effectiveness is not always achievable by individual hospitals in the NHS:

1. Optimum economic efficiency requires the availability of sufficient capital, under-capitalisation being a general cause of failure to reduce unit costs in any situation.
2. Hospital managements generally do not have authority to make their own investment decisions, regional hospital boards being constitutionally responsible for fund allocation and for taking local social as well as economic considerations into account. Regional optimisation entails sub-optimisation at hospital management committee level.
3. Individual hospitals must generally operate at their given scales of specific department sizes, even though a larger scale of department might be more cost-effective.
4. Short-term efficiencies may be incompatible with longer-term ones, especially where phased capital expenditures are involved.
5. Increases of efficiency, while resulting in lower unit costs may, by increasing total output, result in total expenditure's exceeding permissible levels.
6. It is impracticable—or at least not considered acceptable—to declare professional staff in the NHS redundant in order to promote lower unit costs (excepting when individuals obligingly retire or commit some heinous offence).
7. There is a lack, at the central level, of a *modus operandi* based on economic principles as distinct from economies.

I do not doubt that Professor Curnow has made allowances for these factors, and that he has in mind other less plausible reasons for low cost-effectiveness in specific situations. The purpose of demonstrating the more plausible reasons for sub-optimal efficiency is to show: that management neurosis can be too facile a diagnosis on which to base a general prescription suitable for all levels of health service administration; and that some of the more obvious methods of achieving cost-effectiveness as practised in the commercial field are not always applicable to the NHS.

While, however, it is not difficult to be an apologist for apparently low cost-effectiveness in many existing hospital situations, a useful distinction may be made between the problems of promoting cost-effectiveness in existing hospitals or hospital departments, and the problems of efficiency-promotion in new hospital planning situations. In the latter case there is much greater potential for on-going, cost-effective management to inject economic principles into decisions relating to capital and revenue investment, selections of optimum economic scales, determination of economic staff/equipment ratios, and establishment of advanced communication systems. Commercial economic experience is far more relevant to the health service, and in particular the hospital, planning situation than the operational one. The differences between the two situations call for different patterns of research programme and different procedural applications.

In the hospital planning situation, considerations of capital expenditure play a much greater role than in the operational situation—some might say too dominant a role. There exists here a small forest of potential econometric research which is at present mainly a playground for architects. The situation is a standing invitation for (i) the establishment of a programme of operational and econometric research to determine the optimum economic scales of all the constituent activities (subsystems) which collectively make up hospital systems, and (ii) the subsequent development of a simple mathematical technique for calculating the mixes of activities which will result in an optimum health service system, taking account of both hospital and community health services.

Mr Beresford's paper, 'Use of Hospital Costs in Planning', and the recent Bonham-Carter Committee Report on the Functions of the District General Hospital, the one positively and the other perhaps negatively, both lend support to the case for a programme of econometric research in the hospital planning field. The requirement at the present point in time is rather for relatively unsophisticated, quantitative analyses than for subtle mathematical models—the objective may be stated to be improved rather than perfect decision-making.

THE SOCIAL ACCOUNTING OF HEALTH

E. M. SUTCLIFFE

Institute of Social and Economic Research, University of York

---

INTRODUCTION

In recent years there has been a growing concern with the rising costs of medical care and with the problem of allocating limited resources not only within the field of health, but between health and other 'social' and private needs. The ability to make rational policy decisions about health activities is dependent on the planner's being made aware not only of the total resources available for health services, but also of the ways in which these resources are made available. Knowledge of the diverse sources of finance for health services may be indispensable to the planner, since at any point in time increased resources may be more readily available from one source than another.

There have been studies of the costs of health, such as those of Abel Smith[1, 2] which are concerned with defining and categorising health costs and relating them to national resources in order to make cross-national comparisons. Any analysis of this kind is based on the assumption that the health sector can be identified in the relevant social accounts in the same way as any other production sector. It is well-known that the application of the usual social accounting conventions in delineating the health sector gives rise to important conceptual and statistical problems. These problems arise particularly when attempts are made to compare health expenditures with national income aggregates.

The purpose of this paper is therefore twofold. Firstly, to suggest a method of analysing financial flows so that the points at which

---

[1] B. Abel-Smith, *Paying for Health Services*, World Health Organisation, Geneva 1963.

[2] B. Abel-Smith, *An International Study of Health Expenditure*, World Health Organisation, Geneva 1967.

decisions are made about resources and their allocation are made apparent. Secondly, this framework should distinguish between flows which represent transfer payments and monetary flows. It is hoped that this will enable some of the difficulties which arise when health and national resources are compared, to be avoided.

The ways in which the production of health differs from other productive activities and the implications of these differences insofar as they affect the basic accounting structure, will be discussed in Section 1. Section 2 will examine some of the problems which arise when considering the relationship between health expenditures and national income aggregates. In Section 3 an attempt will be made to suggest a possible framework for analysing the financial transactions of the health sector. This will follow closely the methods used for the education sector by Peacock, Glennerster and Lavers.[3, 4] Section 4 will give some discussion of an attempt to fit existing data for the U.K. into the proposed accounting framework.

1. THE PRODUCTION OF HEALTH SERVICES

Superficially at least, it would seem possible that a framework which would indicate how health services are produced and financed could be constructed using the usual social accounting techniques. A production account, showing the value of sales and purchases of health, and a capital account, indicating the financing of investment in plant and stocks, could be drawn up. The 'net output' of the health sector could be determined by calculating the difference between total sales and intermediate purchases.

Attempts to apply these conventional techniques will not advance very far before many statistical and conceptual difficulties arise. Perhaps the problems that arise in the case of the health sector stem mainly from two factors:

(a) the problem of defining the health sector; and
(b) the fact that, as consumers do not necessarily pay directly for services received and producers may not be responsible for raising their own funds, in some sense the sector is characterised

[3] A. T. Peacock and R. Lavers, 'The Social Accounting of Education', *Journal of the Royal Statistical Society*, Series A, Vol. 129, Part 3, 1966.
[4] A. T. Peacock, H. Glennerster and R. Lavers, *Educational Finance: Its Sources and Uses in the United Kingdom*, London 1969 (Oliver and Boyd).

by a network of financial intermediaries interposed between consumers and producers.

Some of the more important problems which occur will be discussed in this section

Definition of the Health Sector
The first problem which arises in the case of the 'production' of health services is that of defining the 'production boundary'. In this instance it is not possible to use the convention of delimiting the sector according to an output 'health' since it is difficult to find an unambiguous definition of 'health'. The use, of say, the World Health Organisation definition of health as "... a state of physical, mental and social well-being and not merely the absence of disease or infirmity" will lead to the necessity of imputing the costs of an element of 'health' which arises as an incidental effect of activities not primarily concerned with the production of health services. Thus it would involve examination of expenditures for such disparate activities as slum clearance, food production and recreation. Further-more, no clear dividing line can be drawn between traditional health services and substitutes for these from such quasi-medical practitioners as chiropractors, herbalists, etc.

It is, however, necessary to at least find a definition of health services which can be consistently applied both through time and in cross-national studies. To some extent the definition of the 'production boundary' is a 'non-problem' since we can adopt the view that health services '... mean just what I choose it to mean—neither more nor less'. Clearly, the definition of health services must include the traditional services such as hospital care, services of physicians, dental care, drugs and public health facilities. Whether or not we include certain fringe activities will remain a matter for controversy, but provided this is made explicit it will be possible to make consistent comparisons with other studies. Whatever definition of health services is adopted, care should be taken to include health activities within branches of government other than health, e.g. medical care for the armed services and school health programmes.

Finally, it should be noted that even if we can arrive at a 'working' definition of health services, certain statistical problems may remain. If a strictly 'economic' definition is used, then imputations of the value of home nursing, services of voluntary agencies, etc. would have to be calculated. To some extent, omission of such imputations can be justified on the grounds that such services are excluded from the national income accounts. A further problem is that of allocating joint costs between 'health' and 'non-health' activities of health institutions. Hospitals, in particular, provide not only medical care but also teaching and research facilities, and may provide such things as accommodation for staff and education for children in their care as well. This raises serious complications in deciding not only allocation of capital but also current costs between various activities.

Organisation and Financing of the Health Sector

An examination of the ways in which health care can be provided and financed shows that the methods of organisation vary greatly from one country to another.[5, 6] Health services can be *provided* by government agencies (both central and local), philanthropic institutions, private profit- and non-profit-making 'health' firms and individual health practitioners. The financial structure of different health services is equally varied except insofar as public health facilities are concerned, which because of indivisibilities, are in general within the sphere of government and financed through taxation. The methods of financing 'personal health' care are perhaps influenced by attempts on the part of individuals and institutions to mitigate the costs to the consumer of a 'catastrophic' episode of ill health. This has led to the growth of health insurance schemes both private and government, to the provision of health facilities by government at zero or near-zero cost to the consumer, financed through taxation, and to the provision of funds and/or facilities by philanthropic institutions. The relative importance of these institutions will vary from one country to another but perhaps these 'indirect' methods of paying for health care are of more significance than any 'fee for service' method, particularly for long-term and costly episodes of illness.

The major problems that arise stem from government intervention in the health sector. The amount and nature of government intervention in either providing and/or financing health services will

[5] O. Anderson, 'Towards a Framework for Analysing Health Services', *Social and Economic Administration*, vol. 1, No. 1, 1967.

[6] M. Seham, 'An American Doctor looks at eleven Foreign Health Systems', *Social Science & Medicine*, vol. 3, No. 1, 1969.

clearly affect not only the total resources available but also the allocation of those resources within the field of health. From a statistical point of view, government control over health services facilitates the collection of data because of the concentration of production in one organisation, but it unfortunately raises serious conceptual problems.

If government participation in health care was restricted to producing and selling 'health', then the presentation of the data would create no problems. Health services, so provided, could be treated as a nationalised industry and incorporated in the production sector in the conventional way. Government intervention complicates the situation, particularly since it can occur in so many ways. It can consist of one or a combination of any of the following: tax relief on medical expenses; grants (capital or current) and loans to private health institutions; or provision of part of all health facilities to some or all consumers at zero or near-zero cost to the consumer.

The intervention of government between provider and user of health services, insofar as it provides subsidies, means that the 'price' of such services is not determined by the usual market mechanism. The resources made available and the quantity of services offered respond more to a complex of political and social forces than to market forces. In these circumstances it is difficult to attach meanings to such notions as 'cost' or 'net output' of health.

A subsidiary point to be considered is that of indirect subsidisation in the private sector through tax concessions. Individual medical expenses may be tax-deductible. Also, voluntary health institutions may be exempt from certain taxes and donations to those institutions may be tax-free. There are basically two problems which arise in attempting to assess the effects of tax concessions. Firstly there is the statistical problem of calculating taxes 'not paid'. The second problem is that private sector resources and the use of those resources are dependent on these concessions being made available, and to include them would involve some double counting.

A final point which should be considered is the effect of philanthropic organisations. Traditionally, philanthropy has provided health facilities and funds in an attempt to moderate the effects of the market. Under certain circumstances this may involve not only financial assistance to medical institutions but donations of services free of charge, e.g. nursing services by religious orders, surgeons who operate without receiving a fee. This raises the problem of the necessity of imputing a value for these professional voluntary services. It should be noted that if a value for these services is imputed, the value of the GNP will also have to be adjusted in the interests of consistency.

Further discussions of the implications of government financing and provision of health care, though providing the most difficult problems in devising a set of simple social accounts, will be given in Section 2. At this point it will be noted that, where subsidisation is of importance and indirect payment common, as with health, it is essential that the financial flows are made explicit in any set of accounts. If this is done then perhaps it will be apparent where the decisions about quantity and allocation of funds are made.

2. HEALTH EXPENDITURE AND NATIONAL INCOME
AGGREGATES

National income can be regarded as the 'money value of goods and services becoming available to the nation' and can be derived in three ways. From the production side we can aggregate *either* the net output of individual industries (national product) *or* factor income (national income). From the consumption aspect the sum of purchases of final output can be calculated (national expenditure). Though it is well-recognised that many problems arise in defining these aggregates, particular difficulty inheres in attempts to analyse the contribution of the health sector to national resources.

As was noted in the previous section, many problems in attempting to evaluate health expenditure arise from the intervention of government and philanthropic institutions between consumers and producers of health services, i.e. the 'price' of health services is not simply the result of the usual market forces. This arises particularly when it is necessary to calculate 'net output' or total expenditure on health. Clearly we cannot legitimately calculate 'net output' of health services by subtracting intermediate inputs from 'total sales' where there is any substantial element of subsidisation, public or private.

From the consumption side we can aggregate purchases by 'final buyers', i.e. households, government and business purchasers of investment goods. Although convention requires that government is a final buyer, it is obvious that in the case of health (as with education) the goods and services purchased are used to produce an output 'health services' which can be valued only in terms of the inputs. The aggregation of government purchases (a measure of inputs) and consumer purchases of health (a measure of output) and comparison with final output, is clearly illegitimate. Even if the alternative course of summing the value of inputs to private and public sectors is followed, inconsistency arises. Private sector purchases of goods and services may comprise not only final goods but also intermediate goods which are not components of final output.

It would appear that the only possible method open to us in the case of the health sector would be to calculate total factor payments: i.e. wages and salaries; rent, interest and profits of private health facilities; imputed rent for public premises; and the imputed value of factor payments for services from 'non-health' firms. This total could then be used as a reasonable measure of the direct costs of health and compared with total factor payments in the economy. Even this procedure is not without snares. Imputation of factor payments, particularly imputed rent of publicly owned property must in essence be fairly arbitrary. Also, since hospitals, for example, do provide certain 'non-health' facilities (teaching, research, staff accommodation, etc.), some statistical difficulty will occur in allocating joint costs.

It should be noted that any estimate of the proportion of national income devoted to health is dependent on the definition chosen. If, for example, we wish to include a value for donated nursing services by religious orders or nursing services provided within the family, then not only do total resources in the health sector increase but a redefinition of national income is necessary.

Even if it is possible to arrive at a valid measure of the proportion of national income spent on health, as suggested above, great care must be taken in making comparisons within a country through time or international comparisons. The effect of increased allocation of resources to the health sector can be measured effectively only if an index of the quantity and quality of health services provided, which is independent of the cost involved, can be developed.

3. FRAMEWORK FOR HEALTH SECTOR ACCOUNTS
Social accounts can be regarded either as a systematic presentation of factual information and/or, perhaps more importantly, as an analytical framework within which certain specific questions may be

answered. Although there is no intention in this section to outline a fully articulated set of social accounts, the framework will conform insofar as it attempts to systematise information on health finance, so that questions about the allocation of funds within the field of health and between health and other activities, may be answered. It is recognised that no single accounting framework will be ideal for all purposes at all times, but it is hoped that enough detail will be available to allow for a certain amount of rearrangement of the data for limited uses outside the scope of this enquiry.

Basically, this paper is concerned with attempting to design a framework which will enable answers to be given to two questions which are of interest to planners and policy-makers within the field of health.

1. What are the total resources absorbed in the health sector compared with resources available in the economy as a whole?
2. What are the relative 'outputs' of private and public health sectors and what are the sources of their funds?

Attention will be concentrated on the second question since our primary concern is for information about the financing of health expenditure. In this section a brief outline of the model accounts for this purpose will be given. This follows quite closely the framework used for education by Peacock, Glennerster and Lavers.[7]

Perhaps the most simple model of the health sector would comprise two parts: (i) a public sector (possibly restricted entirely to public health facilities) financed completely from taxation, and (ii) a private sector (all personal health care facilities) financed entirely by individual households on a 'fee for services' basis. Unfortunately, the situation in the health sector is infinitely more complex since direct payment by individuals for personal health care tends to be the exception rather than the rule. In no country is medical care provided by the private sector alone. Certain public health facilities will be provided by local authorities. In addition, hospital and clinics may be made available for special groups within the community, e.g. the indigent poor and veterans. It is necessary not only to compare the size of each sector financed in different ways but also to analyse the sources of funds for each sector.

The starting point for the accounts will be to set up an expenditure

[7] A. T. Peacock, H. Glennerster and R. Lavers, *op. cit.*

Table 1. Institutional Classification of Expenditure by Domestic Users of Funds

—	Public Health	Personal Health Care						
		Hospitals	Health Centres and Clinics	Physicians	Dental Care	Ophthalmists etc.	Pharma-ceutical Services	Other
Central Government Institutions								
Local Authorities Institutions								
Private Health Institutions								

account for the health sector. This account will be divided into three sub-sectors: health institutions under direct control of central government, local authority facilities and privately organised health facilities. It will be necessary at this point to give some definition of health services since if valid comparisons are to be made the nature of expenditure must be standardised as far as possible. Health services will be defined narrowly to include traditional facilities such as hospitals, services of physicians, services of 'professions supplementary to medicine' such as dentists, ophthalmists, pharmacists, etc., the regulatory and supervisory activities of public health authorities, plus environmental measures aimed at the control of specific diseases.

It is obvious that further subdivision of expenditure is necessary if this information is to be of use to policy-makers. The choice of classification will be to a large extent dependent on the use for which the data is intended and to a much lesser extent on the availability of the data. The possible divisions are numerous but only two examples will be given here. Expenditure could be divided between public and personal health care with further categories within personal health care to distinguish hospitals from clinics, physician services, etc., i.e. an *institutional* classification (see Table 1). Alternatively, a *functional* classification of expenditure could be made in order to isolate 'health expenditure proper'. In this case administration, research and 'non-health expenditure' would be kept separate (see Table 2).

A further subdivision of the data classified in either of these ways

Table 2. Functional Classification of Expenditure by Domestic Users of Funds

—	Administration	Medical Care	Research	Non-health Expenditure
Central Government Institutions				
Local Authority Institutions				
Private Health Institutions				

is suggested should it be intended to calculate health's share of national income. If, as suggested in Section 2, the only legitimate comparison is factor payments in the health sector with total factor payments in the rest of the economy, a subdivision by *economic* category must be made. Thus wages and salaries; rent, interest and profits of private health institutions; imputed rent for public premises, must be abstracted. In principle, this classification is fairly easy to incorporate into the model accounts, but serious problems may be raised when any attempt to obtain and fit data into this scheme is made.

The next step in the procedure is to draw up a revenue account to balance the expenditure account and analyse the sources of funds for each sector. The institutions whether government or private who provide the health services, termed 'receivers of funds', obtain funds from a variety of sources and of various kinds. They may receive fees from individuals (these could be classified as purchases by households), grants from either central or local public authorities, grants from philanthropic institutions and loans from government or enterprises such as banks. These last organisations may be termed 'spending bodies'. The situation is further complicated in the public sector, since, though the Ministry of Health or local health department are 'spending bodies', they are not in general responsible for raising their own funds. Usually, funds are 'allocated' to them by finance departments in central and local government. These bodies will be termed 'allocators of funds'. In turn the 'allocators' obtain their funds from taxes paid by households and enterprises, the 'source of funds'. Even though it is not possible to represent all flows, Table 3 attempts to give some idea of the transactions involved in the health sector.

Perhaps one or two features of Table 3 require clarification. Firstly, since it is not possible to represent all possible flows in diagrammatic form it is necessary to show the detailed flows as a series of matrices; Tables 4, 5 and 6 show movement of funds from sources to allocators, allocators to spending bodies and finally between spending bodies and receivers of funds. It should be noticed that movement of funds occurs both vertically and horizontally. Funds may be 'allocated' by central government to local authority finance departments who then reallocate these funds to health and other departments. Finally, it should be noted that certain transactions are entirely nominal (marked intra-sector transfers in Table 3).

Table 3. Flow of Funds

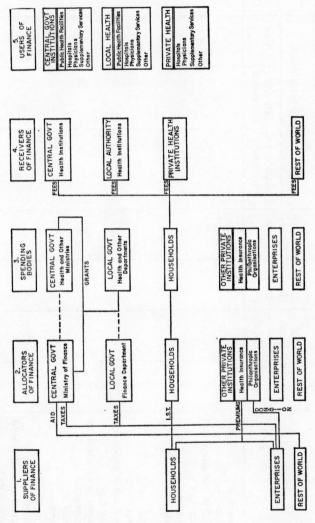

Table 4. Supply of Funds to Allocators

	Government Financial Dept.		House-holds	Enter-prises	Other Private Institutions			Rest of World
—	Central	Local			Philanthropic Institutions	Health Insurance	Other	
Household								
Taxes								
Purchases of goods and services								
Transfers								
Loans								
Enterprises								
Taxes								
Purchases of goods and services								
Interest and dividend payments								
Transfers								
Loans								
Rest of World								
Interest and dividend payments								
Transfers								
Loans								

Table 5. Allocation of Funds of Spending Bodies

| | Central Govt. | | Local Govt. | | House-hold | Enter-prises | Other Private Institutions | Rest of World |
	Ministry of Health	Other Ministries	Health Dept.	Other Dept.				
Central Government								
Grants								
Loans								
Transfers								
Local Government								
Grants								
Loans								
Transfers								
Households								
Transfers								
Enterprises								
Grants								
Loans								
Transfers								
Other Private Institutions								
Transfers								
Loans								
Rest of World								
Transfers								

Table 6. Receipts from Spending Bodies

	Central Govt. Health Institutions	Local Govt. Health Institutions	Private Health Institutions	Rest of World
1. *Central Government*				
(a) *Ministry of Health*				
Grants				
Purchases of goods and services				
Loans				
(b) *Other Ministries*				
Categories as above				
2. *Local Government*				
(a) *Health Department*				
Grants				
Purchases of goods and services				
Loans				
(b) *Other Departments*				
Categories as above				
3. *Households*				
Purchases of goods and services				
Loans				
4. *Other Private Institutions*				
(a) *Philanthropic Trusts*				
Grants				
Purchases of goods and services				
Loans				
(b) *Health Insurance Firms*				
Purchases of goods and services				
Loans				
(c) *Other*				
Grants				
Purchases				
Loans				
5. *Enterprises*				
Grants				
Purchases				
Loans				
6. *Rest of World*				
Categories as above				

It is clear that the household, in paying fees for health facilities, acts as source and allocator of funds as well as spending body. The introduction of these fictitious flows in the scheme, though to some extent unsatisfactory, is perhaps a price which must be paid in order to achieve a consistent analysis of the complex of transactions in the health sector.

Although this framework will lead to an elucidation of the financial transactions and decision-making procedure in the health sector, the rather formalistic analysis will give rise to certain statistical problems. Apart from the lack of easily available data for the private sector, at all stages, major difficulties will arise in obtaining information about transfers between 'source of funds' and 'allocator', and 'allocator' and 'spending bodies'. These problems arise for two main reasons: (i) taxes are rarely earmarked for health services and in consequence it is impossible to associate particular taxes of taxpayers with financing health; (ii) government borrowing is associated with only general expenditure and not specified items of expenditure.

In any attempt to fit specific data into this framework, other problems will inevitably emerge. A discussion follows of some problems involved in an attempt to fit preliminary data for the U.K. into this framework.

4. STATISTICAL SOURCES FOR THE UNITED KINGDOM
Since the data is incomplete at this stage it would perhaps be both inappropriate and misleading to give specific results for the U.K. It is hoped that these results can be made available in due course. Nevertheless some discussion of the data required, its sources and some of the problems encountered will be made in this final section.

It is clear that there are serious gaps in the data in the private sector at all stages. Difficulties in the public sector arise mainly because of the absence of information about transfers between 'source of funds' and 'allocators', and between 'allocators' and 'spending bodies'. In addition a certain amount of reclassification of published data will be required for the public sector. A list of published sources of data is given in the Appendix. Others may be able to suggest other sources, particularly in the private sector.

As suggested by the analysis in Section 3, starting with expenditure in the public and private sectors an attempt will be made to assess the accessibility of data necessary to highlight the transactions from source of funds to final use in the health sector. A brief examination of the data will be made under four subheadings: (i) Expenditure, (ii) Finance of Expenditure by Spending Bodies, (iii) Allocators of Funds to Spending Bodies, and (iv) Suppliers of Funds to Allocators of Finance.

Expenditure

Perhaps it is not surprising that expenditure figures for health services in the public sector, as seen for example in the Central Statistical Office National Income Expenditure (1969) Table 5, are restricted to those services under the auspices of the Ministry of Health and Social Security. This figure for total expenditure (£1,687 million in 1968) suffers from some deficiencies which can fortunately be corrected from other sources. In particular it excludes health facilities under the control of ministries other than Health, especially medical care for the armed services and school health services. Also care must be taken to exclude expenditure on 'non-health' activities included in figures for the NHS, e.g. staff accommodation, canteens, farms and gardens, etc.

The private sector is characterised in official statistics by its absence. The only official estimates appear within the category 'other services' in the National Income and Expenditure estimate of consumer expenditure, but these amounts (about £40 million in 1966) are subject to serious sampling errors.[8] An extensive review of the private sector in England and Wales[9] reports: '. . . There is no accurate reporting of those engaged in private practice, the number of private patients or the income from private practice . . .'. Figures for the number of beds available in private health institutions are given in *The Hospitals Year Book*.[10] A further omission is purchases of drugs in the private sector, largely self-medication, estimated at £79 million in 1966 by the Office of Health Economics.[11] In order to obtain accurate information on the finance of the private sector, returns would be required from all private hospitals and nursing homes and from individual practitioners.

[8] Central Statistical Office, *National Accounts Statistics, Sources and Methods*, 1968 (H.M.S.O.).
[9] S. Mencher, *British Private Medical Practice and the National Health Service*, Pittsburg 1968 (University of Pittsburgh Press).
[10] The Institute of Hospitals Administrators, *The Hospitals Year Book*, 1969.
[11] Office of Health Economics, *Without Prescription*, London 1968.

Finance of Expenditure by Spending Bodies

The spending bodies concerned in financing health are departments and ministries of health, other government departments and ministries, households, enterprises and other private institutions. In each case it is necessary to distinguish between grants, purchases and loans.

The majority of financial transactions in the public sector are national, i.e. grants from central or local government. Certain direct payments, purchases, are made by households to institutions within the NHS, e.g. fees for dental treatment, prescription charges and payment for amenity beds in hospitals. In addition, fees are charged to private patients for the use of accommodation within NHS hospitals. Additional finance is available from the Hospital Endowments Fund.

In the private sector, information is very slight except where health insurance firms like BUPA are involved. Estimates are required for direct payments by patients to private health institutions and private practitioners. Also, information is required on loans from such institutions as banks and on grants from charitable organisations.

Allocation of Funds to Spending Bodies

At this stage of the analysis the case of households and enterprises is of little interest. For the most part notional transfers occur from, for example, households conceived of as allocators to households conceived of as spending bodies.

The distinction between allocator and spending body is perhaps of most significance in the case of local authorities. Local health departments incur expenditure but are not responsible for raising their own funds. Specific grants are not given by central government nor are specific taxes raised by local authorities to finance health. The contribution of central government to local authority expenditure is mainly through the General Grant, which contributes to a range of services; these include not only health but such things as education, welfare services, etc. The remainder of local health department expenditure will be financed through the rates. The problem which arises is to determine the proportion of health expenditure which is financed from the General Grant and the proportion financed from the rates.

Suppliers of Funds to Allocators of Finance

The final suppliers of funds are households, enterprises and the rest of the world. Funds are made available through taxes paid to central government, rates paid to local authorities and donations to philanthropic institutions. Though income tax and surtax can be regarded as transfers from households to government and profits tax as transfers by enterprises, the proportion of indirect taxation paid by households and enterprises is impossible to determine. Similar problems arise in determining the proportions of rate income attributable to households and enterprises respectively.

Finally, little information is available in easily accessible form about the income of philanthropic institutions.

ACKNOWLEDGEMENTS

Thanks are due to The Nuffield Provincial Hospital Trust for a grant to enable this work to be done. Thanks are also due to Professor A. T. Peacock for many helpful suggestions and discussions.

APPENDIX

A certain amount of summarised information is available from:

Central Statistical Office, *National Income and Expenditure*, Tables, London (H.M.S.O.).

Department of Health and Social Security, *Digest of Health Statistics for England and Wales*, London (H.M.S.O.).

Central Statistical Office, *Family Expenditure Survey*, London (H.M.S.O.).

More detailed information based on and supplementing the Appropriation Accounts can be found in the following:

Summarised accounts (separately for England and Wales and Scotland).

Regional Hospital Boards, Boards of Governors of Teaching Hospitals, Hospital Management Committees, Executive Councils and Dental Estimates Board (House of Commons Paper (H.C.)), London (H.M.S.O.).

Hospital Endowments Fund (H.C.), London (H.M.S.O.).

Summary of Health Services Accounts (N. Ireland) (H.C.), London (H.M.S.O.).

Local Governmental Financial Statistics (England and Wales), London (H.M.S.O.).

Local Financial Returns (Scotland), London (H.M.S.O.).

Local Authority Financial Returns (N. Ireland), London (H.M.S.O.).

COMMENT ON 'THE SOCIAL ACCOUNTING OF HEALTH'

D. S. LEES
University of Nottingham

In commenting on papers I generally ask myself three questions: What is the author attempting to do? Has the author succeeded in doing it? and Is it worth doing?

In relation to the first question, although Mrs Sutcliffe states her purpose clearly, an explicit recognition of the fundamental truth that national income data are *a measure of economic welfare* would clarify her discussion. Goods are made for people and not people for goods: this is the essential value-judgement of social accounting.

Mrs Sutcliffe discusses the problem of the 'output' of health services, but she does not resolve it. It is not only that we lack market prices for health services that can be interpreted at least as rough indicators of consumer preferences, so that aggregation can be carried out in a way consistent with the rest of the aggregation procedure in the national accounts; it is also that this 'output' is not easily defined to enable health expenditures to be divided into 'consumption' and 'investment'. These problems are very important nowadays since zero-price goods and services supplied by the government now account for about 20% of national income.

We are thus confronted with a paradox: social accounting becomes more useful as markets are used less. But the social accounts also *mean* less as the non-market area expands.

These seem to me to be some of the fundamental difficulties in the social accounting of zero-price goods and services. Others mentioned by Mrs Sutcliffe on p. 240 are *not* peculiar to health, but are common to a wide range of goods and services.

The author has been successful in what she set out to do, but her success has been at the cost of raising major conceptual problems: in particular, how to interpret the numbers that she will doubtless be putting into her little boxes. There is no difficulty in accumulating social accounting data and arranging it into all manner of patterns. Research work could go on forever along these lines. The basic question is, what (if anything) does any particular pattern mean and how do we choose between patterns?

Regarding the usefulness of the exercise, I suppose that such data could be useful to the Department of Health and Social Security, which might be able to use shares in GNP as part of a case for more spending on health. Moreover, in isolating an 'investment' component, there is some basis for rate of return calculations, cost-benefit calculations and other efficiency exercises of relevance to planning the future quantities of human and non-human resources devoted to medical care. Systematical international comparisons of GNP proportions spent on health, if performed in a consistent and comprehensive manner, may also shed interesting light on the activity of governments in different countries and show how total spending on health varies internationally.

However, at this level of aggregation, I do not see how the information can be useful to decision-makers *within* the health field, where economic expertise is probably most fruitfully applied. For this purpose, a more detailed definition of the 'health industry' would be useful to planners. An extension of the ideas outlined on p. 240 of Mrs Sutcliffe's paper might, in this respect, provide the most promising avenue for future work in this area. Ultimately, the practical problems to be solved are of a micro, not a macro, nature.

Chapter VI

INTERNATIONAL STUDIES

ON THE ECONOMIC ANALYSIS OF HEALTH AND MEDICAL CARE IN A SWEDISH HEALTH DISTRICT

J.-E. SPEK

School of Economics and Business Administration, and University of Gothenburg, Sweden.

INTRODUCTION

Against the background of the rising costs of medical care and successively heavier taxation for medical uses coupled with a permanent shortage of personnel, two main questions are raised in Sweden today:

1. How great and of what type is the morbidity in different regions in the country (extent, causes, effects)?
2. How can medical care be allocated in the most desirable way?

In Sweden some research on these questions is beginning. The aim of this paper is twofold:

1. To present some tentative general definitions within a theoretical framework to serve as a necessary conceptual instrument when disentangling the problem area, and to formulate the relevant questions to guide the more detailed analysis of health and disease. In this conceptual apparatus the factors of knowledge and valuation are introduced from the beginning, which would seem to be necessary for a fruitful positive as well as normative analysis, and it is hoped that the apparatus is broad enough to be understandable for both economists and medical experts and therefore useful for inter-disciplinary research.
2. To report on a planned research project in a Swedish health district named Dalby.

HEALTH AND MEDICAL CARE: DEFINITIONS

The following are the main components in the system of health and medical care:

(1) *Public health care*: those activities which are directly and mainly aimed at the healthy individual, the aim of which is to prevent disease and promote health and well-being. This definition comprises both constructive and preventive measures. Public health can be divided into:

(a) Environmental care: those activities aimed at shaping the external physical and biological conditions for better health; and
(b) personal preventive care: those activities directly aimed at individuals or groups, e.g. health controls, health consultations and vaccinations.

(2) *Medical care*: those activities which are mainly and directly aimed at the sick individual, and of which the aim is, by diagnosis and therapy, to diagnose and cure the sickness and bring about normal biological and social functioning. Medical care can be divided into:

(a) medical care in the strict sense: those activities which are directly aimed at the disease and/or organ, and of which the aim is to give radical or at least symptomatic treatment; and
(b) convalescent care and rehabilitation: those activities which mostly take place after medical care in the strict sense, and of which the aim is not to cure the sickness or palliate the symptoms, but to bring about best possible functioning and ability to work.

ON MULTIFACTORIAL ETIOLOGY

A certain individual's endowment with health and capacity are determined through time by both factors beyond control (Box I in Figure 1) and factors under varying degrees of control by the individual himself and/or society (Boxes II and III).

Consider a certain individual characterised as healthy at point of time t_0. His endowment and capacity will constitute a certain degree of adaptability in relation to changes among the factors in Box II. The development of the individual's state of health after t_0 will depend on the changes among the factors in Box II (constellation and speed of the changes) in relation to his endowment and capacity (which of course in turn are affected by his ageing). Balance must be maintained if the individual is to remain healthy. There are very complicated causal relations between the factors in Box II, and between these and the individual. Two examples of possible sequential events are:

1. Healthy person aged 55→working-place goes into liquidation

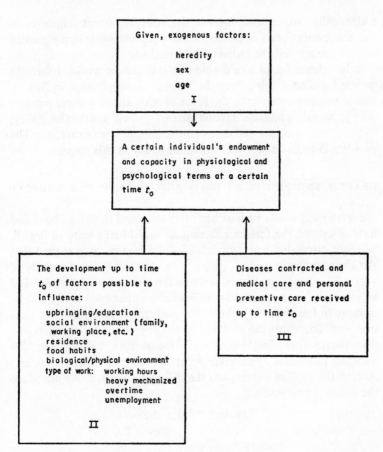

Figure 1. Factors Determining an Individual's Endowment with Health and Capacity

→a new job with lower wage→inferior food and residence→sickness→permanently deficient capacity→new work with still lower wage→social relief measures→etc. (vicious circle).
2. Healthy well-educated person→interesting work and good income →ability to make use of health information, health controls, etc. →ageing brings still better work→etc. (self-reinforcing positive sequence of events).

State of health, working conditions, income, etc. affect each other reciprocally. We seek to discover the most important sequences of the above-mentioned kind, and what their economic consequences are for society and the individual respectively.

If imbalance looks like developing this can be avoided through public influences being brought to bear on the factors in Box II. Public measures may take the form of educational policy, incomes policy, social insurance, labour market policy, residential policy, social care, environmental care or personal preventive care, etc. The problem is to build an efficient overall policy in this respect.

HEALTH AND SICKNESS: NEED AND DEMAND FOR MEDICAL CARE

We have used words such as health, disease and sickness above and have discussed the factors affecting an individual's state of health. Without discussing here any definitions of 'health', it is argued that the characterisation of an individual's state of health in terms of varying degrees of health and sickness is a question of knowledge and valuation. We can say that an individual is either completely healthy or more or less sick. Let us here disregard the varying degrees of sickness and introduce the dichotomy healthy/sick. Now we imagine three parties answering 'yes' or 'no' to the question 'sick?' concerning a certain individual at a certain point of time. The three parties are: society, the medical experts and the individual himself. We introduce the following notation.

Party:	*Answer:*	
	Yes	No
Society	S	$\bar{S}$
Medical experts	M	$\bar{M}$
Individual	I	$\bar{I}$

We assume that society and the medical experts make their judgements and give their answer on the basis of perfect information on the state of health of the individual, i.e. disregarding diagnostic difficulties etc. The individual is assumed to answer on the basis of subjective symptoms and other information that he may have at the time.

If an individual becomes sick (or injured), then the sickness may be such that it is: self-curing, impossible to cure (but usually relief can be given) or possible to cure in varying degrees through influence of the factors in Box II and/or through medical care. If the sickness can be cured or relief be given and this is not to take place through the influence of the factors in Box II (exclusive of food habits), then there is *need* of medical care (including dietary consultation). Depending on the type of sickness, the individual, etc. the need can be satisfied by: the individual himself, laymen (family and friends), or publicly or privately run institutions for medical care. The first two are called self-care and the last public care. Again all this is a question of knowledge and valuation, and we can combine the question 'sick?' with the question 'need for public care?' and let the three parties give a yes/no answer as before.

Finally the demand concept is introduced. *Demand* (active, effective) for public care is that part of the need for care which is represented by those individuals who come in touch with the system of public care with a desire for consultation and treatment, and who are willing to wait if this cannot be provided at once. In each period, demand takes the form of queueing or results in *consumption* (i.e. satisfied demand). We can combine the two above-mentioned questions with a yes/no indication of whether demand is assumed to result or not.

Figure 2 shows the more interesting possible configurations of the various yes/no replies. Case 1 represents *justified* demand with society and medical experts in agreement. Cases 2, 3 and 11 represent *latent need* with society and medical experts in agreement. Cases 5, 6, 8, 9, 12 and 13 represent latent need with society and medical experts in disagreement. Cases 10 and 14 represent *unjustified* demand with society and medical experts in agreement. Cases 4 and 7 represent demand with society and medical experts in disagreement.

As mentioned, the answers to the first and second questions depend on knowledge and valuation, but they offer quite different educational and informational problems; this in turn will affect the ease with which the latent need in the different cases can be converted to demand, as well as unjustified demand be suppressed. Latent need may also be defined as need together with absence of demand for public care. It is partly known through population studies and from individuals who, having contacted the system of public care, have refused to wait. This is not the place to discuss the problems which arise when society and medical experts are in disagreement on latent need. If Case 4 is regarded as justified active demand, then it represents the thorny problem of how to have the doctors furnish the

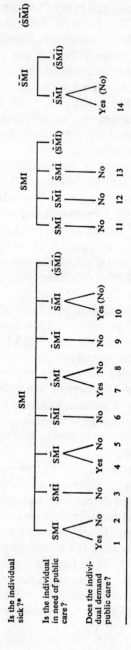

Is the individual sick?*

| | | SMI | | | | SMI | | | | SMI | | | | $\overline{SMI}$ |

Is the individual in need of public care?

| SMI | | SMĪ | | SM̄I | | SM̄Ī | | SMI | | SMĪ | | SM̄I | | SM̄Ī |

Does the individual demand public care?

| SMI | | SMĪ | | SM̄I | | SM̄Ī | | SMI | | SMĪ | | SM̄I | | (SM̄Ī) | | SMI | | SMĪ | | SM̄I | | (SM̄Ī) |

| Yes | No | No | Yes | No | No | Yes | Yes (No) | No | No | No | Yes (No) |
| 1 | 2 | 3 | 4 | 5 | 6 | 7 | 8 | 9 | 10 | 11 | 12 | 13 | 14 |

* The four cases S̄MI, S̄MĪ, S̄M̄I and S̄M̄Ī are disregarded in spite of their great interest. They must not be forgotten in a more detailed analysis. In addition we do not discuss differences in agreement among representatives of society and among medical experts.

Figure 2. Health and Sickness: Need and Demand for Medical Care

right care. If Case 7 is regarded as unjustified demand, it represents the thorny problem of 'over-use'.

As soon as we recognise that medical care is not some sort of homogeneous commodity but consists of a great many activities of different types, qualities and quantities, and that the activities can be combined in different ways, it is evident that the above conceptual scheme has to be much refined and extended. We shall not embark on this here for the intention has only been to propose a medical-economic skeleton of concepts useful for unified medical-economic research concerning health and medical care. The most important thing is that the conceptual scheme is thought-provoking and gives rise to relevant questions by identifying possible conflicts and problems clearly.

Some important general questions are stated below where the conceptual scheme in a refined and extended form may be of help in specifying the appropriate questions and suggesting interesting hypotheses. For example: How large is the need for community care and how is it composed? Which factors are determining the demand for public care, and in what way and to which extent (state of health, valuation, knowledge, information, income, prices, insurance, travelling possibilities, etc.)? How is the consumption of public care determined through the interplay of the demand for and supply of care? Which factors affect absence from work? Which factors affect utilisation of sickness insurance? Is the system of public care functioning efficiently, viewed against the background of prevailing latent need and demand, knowledge of possible treatments and the costs of treatment? If not, how can efficiency be raised?

Economic research can contribute to the answering of these important questions. Demand analysis and welfare economics are especially relevant. It is evident that the answers to all these questions and all the resulting further questions imply the analysis of very complicated causal relations. Such analysis will be possible only through co-operation between medical, economic and social researchers. It is also evident that the analysis presupposes continuing and comprehensive data gathering. The Swedish town of Dalby offers an opportunity for exploring the feasibility of this on an experimental level.

THE DALBY HEALTH DISTRICT

Dalby is a community of about 8,500 people situated 10–20 km from the towns of Malmö and Lund. Since February 1968 the National Board of Health and Welfare and the regional health authority have run a modern centre for personal preventive care, medical care and research on new diagnostic and therapeutic techniques and on the morbidity of the population. A key feature is the fast introduction of the new research findings into clinical use. Two more key features are continuing health controls and dispensaries, and comprehensive gathering of data on each inhabitant, concerning not only consultations, hospitalisation and drug consumption but also education, income, work, etc. In addition, two comprehensive investigations into the state of the mental health of the population were undertaken in the 1940s and 1950s. One thing more must be mentioned: the team of researchers (hitherto mainly medical) work in close co-operation.

The most interesting feature of Dalby is the opportunities it offers for a penetrating dynamic analysis, on the micro-level, of the state of health of the population and the working of the system of public health and medical care. The intention is to start economic research of this kind in Dalby in July 1970. The research will be of a positive as well as a normative kind, and the general aim is to contribute to the answering of the questions posed above.

FRENCH STUDIES ON HEALTH ECONOMICS: A SURVEY

M. E. LEVY

Ministère de la Santé Publique et de la Sécurité Sociale, Paris, France

INTRODUCTION

The economic approach to health problems is a very recent development in France, having been systematically used only since 1960. Before this time only doctors or administrators were concerned with the health system.

Economists have chiefly been concerned with the fast growth of health expenditure and the problems of financing the health care system, faced by social security institutions. They have concentrated on the rational allocation of resources in this area.

The elaboration of the fourth Plan and especially the fifth (1965–1970), which included the health system's development in the total programme of the French economy, gave rise to a number of studies that would not have otherwise appeared. Health statistics have been regularly gathered only from that time. Previously, only approximate administrative evaluations were provided. These statistics, however, are still not sufficient because of the lack of funds allocated to the official services in charge. Real economic studies have been the concern only of private agencies (SEMA, AUROC, CEGOS, etc.). However, these studies have progressively been developed in: research institutions financed by public funds (CREDOC, CEPREMAP), the civil service itself (Ministry of Health and Ministry of Finance) and also at universities (as doctoral dissertations and more rarely as collective research programmes). These studies have focussed on three important subjects: needs and demand, factors influencing costs and supply, and choice criteria for health policy.

NEEDS AND DEMAND

In this section I shall outline some of the different studies based on the various views that different scholars have taken of these needs.

'Real' Needs

Concerning 'real' needs of the population (which we must distinguish from the 'felt' needs and 'expressed' needs), the only study existing in France has been made by INSERM[1] on a sample of 1,500 families representing the population of Soissons in the Aisne. The enquiry was directed toward households in order to study their real needs and the level of the satisfaction of these needs, as well as toward official agencies in order to measure the adequacy of their performance relative to the population's needs.

The purpose of the enquiry was to establish a needs hierarchy. The factors to be taken care of were the numerical importance of registered diseases and the consequences of these diseases on the individuals themselves (on their lives as well as on their living conditions and their professional activity) and on society in general. There were two conclusions:

1. Some special diseases (respiratory, digestive diseases and accidents) all present serious consequences from different points of view: high incidence, high mortality risk, important disturbances for the individual and wider consequences for society.
2. Some other diseases do not present all these characteristics, e.g. there is a low rate of interruptions in education for cardiovascular and for mental diseases; a low rate of mortality but important functional disturbances for the individual and the collectivity in osteo-articular diseases; and there are minor social consequences and negligible mortality but numerous and serious functional disturbances for dental diseases.

From the study on measures used by official services it appears that the main aspects of inadequacy in meeting these needs result from three factors:

(a) the fact that official services are concerned only with a few health problems: protection against some infectious diseases (e.g. TB) or against mental illness; but very important problems which need preventive and educational action that would be immediately profitable, are not taken into account, e.g. road accidents, dental diseases and nutrition problems;

[1] INSERM (Institut National de la Santé et de la Recherche Médicale), 'Recherches sur les Besoins de Santé d'une Population', *Bulletin de l'INSERM*, No. 3, p. 613, 1969.

(b) an imbalance between preventive and curative activities—it seems that the best approach in this area is an emphasis on preventive care that is integrated into everyday life, e.g. in people's workplaces; and

(c) an absence of co-ordination between the various domiciliary services.

'Instrumental' Needs

Numerous studies on 'instrumental' needs have been prepared by SEMA[2] and especially an attempt to evaluate bed needs for 1975.

The method used was to estimate the value in 1975 of the beds/population index from data concerning the other hospitals' activity indexes. Calling P the population at risk, L the existing number of beds, E the annual hospital admissions, and J the number of occupied bed-days per year, we have:

$$I = 1,000 \, L/P \text{ (bed/population index)}$$
$$f = 1,000 \, E/P \text{ (admission rate)}$$
$$b = (100/365) \, J/L \text{ (bed occupation rate)}$$
$$s = J/E \text{ (average length of stay)}$$

and

$$I = (100/365) \, fs/b$$

On the basis of extrapolations concerning f, b and s to 1975 and of comparisons between these French data and easily available foreign data from the U.S.A., Sweden, etc., an average value for 1975 was obtained. Thus, the bed/population index obtained for general hospitals was 10% greater than that of 1962 because of the compensation between the diminishing stay duration and the rising admission rate.

In 1962 the index was too high for anti-TB institutions and too low in mental illness hospitals. But those estimates did not take into account the quality of beds: the needs for 1975 were expressed in terms of modern beds while in 1962 an important proportion of existing beds were to be replaced. Thus, other studies were set in motion to estimate the availability of public hospital beds, especially for the Paris District in 1963. This study has now shown that 46%

[2] SEMA (Société d'Economie et de Mathématique Appliquées), 'Essai d'Evaluation des Besoins en Equipement Hospitalier en 1975', *Bulletin d'Information du Ministère de la Santé Publique et de la Population, Supplément 'Statistiques'*, No. 1, 1964.

of beds were in buildings more than sixty years old and that in the total area it was impossible to set up more than 50% actual beds according to the theoretical standards implied by the index.

Demand

Medical services demand was the subject of a household enquiry in 1960, repeated in 1968 by CREDOC.[3] It had been possible to measure the influence of different factors on demand. In particular:

Morbidity. The influence of morbidity on medical care consumption has three aspects:

(a) large dispersion of sickness risk: 3% of individuals use $\frac{1}{3}$ of total medical services and 15% use $\frac{2}{3}$ while 50% of the population use only 3% of the whole;

(b) large influence of age: the sickness risk is very high at birth, then diminishes, reaching a minimum between the ages of ten and twenty, then grows exponentially (consumption is three to five times higher for the very young and the very old);

(c) different morbidity according to sex, e.g. at all ages women's medical care demand is higher.

Psychosociological factors. Socio-economic class is the main factor, consumption doubling along the scale. Dwelling-place, urban or rural, explains 70% of the variation in consumption. Educational level has a similar order of effect. The number of persons living at home has a very strong influence: individuals in a two-person family consume twice as much medical care as a five-to-nine person family. These four variables are strongly correlated, however, and they only express the influence of more fundamental factors such as the attention paid to health, the information on medical care possibilities and the time available to visit a doctor.

Economic factors. The income effect on consumption seems very low (the income elasticity varies from 0·06 to 0·7) but is different according to income level and type of medical care (higher for example for dental care). The effect of price and the influence of social insurance systems were also found to be very low. The main factor explaining the growth of expenditure on medical care is

[3] CREDOC (Centre de Recherches et de Documentation sur la Consommation), various articles published in *Consommation*, Annales du CREDOC, Paris, since 1958.

scientific knowledge and technical progress. That is, it appears that medical care demand is governed by supply. Availability and proximity of medical services encourage a higher consumption.

Economic Accounting

Economic accounting on health has begun with some CREDOC and INSEE figures where expenditure is classified according to:

(a) various output categories of the health care system, e.g. ambulatory and domiciliary care, hospital care and medical goods;
(b) financial means: ranging from the social security system, public relief, mutual insurance, to private expenditure;
(c) production sectors: doctors, out-patients departments, public hospitals, private hospitals, laboratories, etc.; and
(d) different kinds of medical care activity: preventive medicine, screening, curative medicine, rehabilitation, medical education, scientific research, administration, etc.

These figures in both physical and monetary terms show the structure of the main health system and are the basis for all projections concerning health expenditure during the next five-year plan. It is thus possible to identify the main difficulties or bottlenecks and the choices which we have to make.

COSTS AND SUPPLY

Studies on costs and supply conditions concern essentially the hospital service.

Cost of Illness

A study on the 'Cost of Illness' was done by AREPA on the basis of surgery department information from the Caen Hospital's surgical department.[4] Diseases were classified into twenty-one homogeneous types and the 'real' cost of each one revealed the enormous cross-subsidisation existing due to the uniform price charged for every day's stay in the surgical department. With a uniform daily price which was 85 F in 1967, the real daily cost varied from 50 to 276 F according to the disease.

[4] AREPA (Association pour la Recherche Pure et Appliquée), *Analyse du Coût de la Maladie dans le Service de Chirurgie de l'Hopital de Caen en 1967*, Ministère des Affaires Sociales, Paris 1968.

The average real cost for each type of disease varied (taking into account the average duration of stay) from 660 to 7,200 F, while for the hospital's accounting the difference was only from 520 to 5,800 F.

This study thus demonstrated, for example, that patients with fractured limbs subsidised the others. It showed again that length of stay is frequently not justified from a medical point of view and is only explained either by social considerations or by the low-quality management in hospitals.

Problem of Size

Several AUROC studies between 1963 and 1966 were focussed on factors explaining hospitals costs and on this basis tried to give an answer to the optimal size problem.[5] Statistical relations between expenditures and the number of patients on the one hand and some hospital activity parameters on the other hand, are established for each type of expenditure separately (administrative, food, wages, medical expenditures). These relations revealed, for example, that:

(a) administrative expenditures for each registered patient and food expenses for each day can be considered as constant with respect to size (85 F and 4 F respectively in 1961);
(b) daily wages are a linear function of duration of stay; and
(c) medical expenditure for each patient in the surgery department is a linear function of the average importance of operations in the department.

In general, the conclusion was that the cost per patient is independent of the hospital's size if the quality of care is constant, that the tariff structure in hospitals prevents all serious evaluation of productivity or profitability, and that the hospitals' prices are not good indicators of management quality.

These results enabled the formulation of a mathematical model relating cost per patient to various hospital activity indexes. Thus, a 10% relative decrease in duration of stay is followed by a 5% medical cost per patient decrease in surgery or general medicine departments, but implies a 5% daily price increase. When the occupation rate

[5] AUROC (Société pour l'Avancement et l'Utilisation de la Recherche Opérationnelle Civile), *La Formation du Coût des Soins Hospitaliers*, Paris 1966.

increases from 70 to 85% the result is a 5% average decrease in medical cost per patient.

All these AUROC studies constitute the basis of a statistical management control system which was experimented with in 1968 in Britain and which will be progressively applied to the whole of France in the next few years.

Occupation Rates

A SEMA research on occupation rates in public hospitals led to a general model for the determination of optimal sizes for departments within hospitals.[6] A mathematical model is first formulated in order to describe a hospital department's operations on the basis of five variables: the average number of daily registered patients; the average duration; of stay the maximum beds number (permanent beds and supplementary beds); the average occupation rate; and the failure index—a new concept—which is the probability that the department shall be full on a given day.

These five variables are linked by two mathematical relations and when three variables are given it is possible to obtain the two others. It is thereby possible:

(a) to fix the department size and occupation rate according to the number of daily registered patients, to an estimated average duration of stay and to a given failure index, and

(b) to determine the working conditions of a given department if the number of beds, the admissions per day and the duration of patients' stay are known.

From the occupation rate and the failure index which can be derived from these data, it is possible to calculate the number of patients refused in a year, the number of refused days and the average number of occupied beds.

The method applied here to a department can be generalised to the whole hospital if its departments are not specialised. It is also possible to calculate the bed surplus for a given failure index.

Other Studies

Finally, it is necessary to mention several monographs on hospitals

[6] SEMA, 'Résultats d'une Etude sur le Coefficient d'Occupation des Hôpitaux Publics', *Bulletin d'Information du Ministère de la Santé Publique et de la Population, Supplément 'Statistiques'*, No. 2, 1965.

prepared in order to give a better view of the production function and greater flexibility in the medical care production system.

CHOICES AND CHOICE CRITERIA FOR A HEALTH POLICY

Most recent French studies on health economics are now focussed on problems concerning choices and choice criteria. This is partially the result of PPBS studies at the U.S. Department of Health, Education and Welfare and partially due to the large programme initiated by the French Ministry of Finance on budgetary choices rationalisation throughout the entire French public administration.

A first methodological paper issued by the Forecasting Department in the Ministry of Finance[7] tried to show in what manner cost-benefit analysis could be adapted to health problems with special application to the setting of fractures. But principally this paper makes clear the types of benefits to take into account and the means of measuring them. These benefits are:

(a) the production benefit (i.e. the recovered economic activity measured through wages);
(b) the well-being benefit (when after-effects of disease are reduced);
(c) the leisure benefit (when illness is shortened or avoided); and
(d) the life benefit (prolongation of life for itself).

Two recent studies tried to apply the method of cost-benefit analysis to TB and mental illness in children.

Tuberculosis

An epidemiological model permits the calculation of the avoided sick number in each period according to the incidence of illness and to the BCG vaccination efficiency rate.[8] Treatment benefits (cost of avoided treatments) and the production benefits are calculated for two distinguished aspects of TB. Taking a 10% prevalence rate, the vaccination generalisation project appears very profitable, the actual net benefit being 100 million F. After that the results are tested according to different parameter values (incidence rate, actualisation rate, etc.).

[7] Ministère de l'Economie et des Finances, Direction de la Prévision, *Note sur les Methodes d'Application de Calculs Coût-Avantages aux Services Hospitaliers*, Paris 1967.

[8] Ministère de l'Economie et des Finances, Direction de la Prévision, *Etude Economique de la Rentabilité de la Vaccination BCG*, Paris 1969.

Mental Illness

The purpose of the mental illness study[9] was to compare the costs and benefits of different organisations of preventive and curative medicine concerning children's mental illness. The first step was to establish an organisation typology according to their more or less complex character, objective and therapeutical techniques, according to staff and equipment arrangements, characteristics of the population at risk, and so on. The cost problem gave rise to no particular difficulties, the benefit problem being the main preoccupation of the study. After having analysed them, three benefit indicators were chosen: a school-life indicator, a family adaptation indicator and a society adaptation indicator.

For each of these indicators different criteria were propounded which enabled the degree of benefit to be estimated, e.g. for the family adaptation indicator there were two criteria: (i) the parent's attitude (1 for normal tolerance, 0·3 for hyperprotection and 0 for rejection), and (ii) the child's attitude (1 for normal, 0·8 for excessive requirements, 0·5 for personality trouble and 0 for hyperaggressivity).

Output Budgeting

A larger output budgeting study is in progress at the Public Health Ministry.[10] The purpose is to compare the costs and benefits of different medical care systems concerning all mentally sick, and especially to evaluate those which derive from the sectorisation policy defined in 1960. This policy implies for each sector staff: responsibility for a whole given population from the point of view of its mental health; continuity and personalisation of care; and the keeping of the patient in his family circle and in his social sphere.

All these features require a large diversification of out-patient departments and medical teams. Using cost-benefit analysis, answers to these questions were sought from this study: Has priority to be given to hospital building or to out-patient care at once with the present stock of resources? How far is it possible to develop—from

[9] Ministére de l'Economie et des Finances, Direction de la Prévision, and Ministère de la Santé Publique et de la Sécurité Sociale, Service des Etudes et des Prévisions, *Etude Coût-Avantages de Deux Organisations de Soins pour les Malades Mentaux Enfants*, Paris 1969.

[10] Ministère de la Santé Publique et de la Sécurité Sociale (Groupe RCB Maladies Mentales), *Note de Présentation de l'Etude de Rationalisation des Choix Budgétaires concernant les Maladies Mentales*, Paris 1969.

the medical and financial points of view—early screening for these patients? Taking into account the fact that medical opinions differ on the most appropriate therapies, does this imply a preference for one or several organisation types over others and why?

The first investigations prove that the main difficulties are psychological and derive from the doctors' failure to admit even the possibility of quantifying any of the benefits, the absence of their co-operation in developing an operational approach, and more general difficulties arising from lack of information.

Screening

A more systematic study according to cost-benefit analysis principles has been done by CEPREMAP on the early screening of cervical cancer.[11] Costs and benefits were measured with regard to a situation in which there is no screening. To this situation is related a medical care demand, an annual expenditures level and cervical cancer mortality rates of each class of age and for each year.

A probabilistic model of the disease's history is then formulated with several illness spells, their duration and the probabilities that one spell develops into another, medical care demand and the survival rates after treatment. The efficiency of a given screening policy was then tested by comparing its costs and benefits. An optimal screening programme was studied for women aged 20 when screening began. This programme implies a four-year test periodicity from the ages of 25 to 60.

The net economic benefit was found to be positive despite a very low value chosen for life (113,000 F) and the profitability rate was 13·5% in constant prices—superior to most of the rates of return found on other investments in the public sector.

Value of Human Life

Different studies have been made on the implicit value of human life based on the costs the community will accept in order to protect it. These show a very large dispersion of implicit prices which vary from 1 to 100. But in the road safety studies the average chosen price is 300,000 F.

---

[11] CEPREMAP (Centre d'Etudes Prospectives d'Economie Mathématique Appliquées à la Planification), *Une Etude Economique de la Prévention et du Depistage Précoce du Cancer du Col de l'Uterus*, Paris 1969.

Recently an official commission has tried for two years to study the long-range evolution factors concerning the health system and to establish the prospects for the future levels of health in the community as a necessary basis for a health policy.[12]

On the basis of the probable demographic, economic, cultural and technical features of society in 1985, the study tried to determine the evolution of needs and how the means must be developed to obtain a more rational and more co-ordinated system in the future. Particular attention was given to the large possibilities offered by an integrated information system in the health area, to the regional distribution of hospitals, to the role of out-patient care, and finally to the future of preventive action of an individual or collective variety.

CONCLUDING REMARKS

All these recent French studies reveal the development of modern thinking about health planning. The simple needs approach is being replaced by the more systematic formulation of objective functions and an analysis of the necessary means of attaining these objectives. A restricted concentration on physical equipment planning is being replaced by a more general approach including the planning of future human resources in more behaviouristic models of the health care system. Finally, more attention is being paid to the efficient use of current resources within the existing framework.

[12] *Réflexions sur l'Avenir du Système de Santé, Contribution à l'Elaboration d'une Politique Sanitaire*, Rapport du Groupe de Travail sur la Prospective de la Santé, La Documentation Française, Paris 1969.

THE ECONOMICS OF HEALTH SERVICES IN THE UNITED STATES

H. R. BOWEN

Chancellor and Professor of Economics, Claremont University Center

and

J. R. JEFFERS

Associate Professor of Economics and Director, Health Economics Research Center, The University of Iowa

INTRODUCTION

The American people are currently in a somewhat agitated frame of mind. They are deeply disturbed and divided by the Vietnamese war, by poverty in the midst of affluence, by the decay of the inner cities, by racial strife and injustice, by environmental pollution, by price inflation, and by the sometimes outrageous behaviour of the young. In addition to all this, they are troubled about the health care system. Its costs are rising astronomically while the quantity and quality of health care and the health of the nation seem not to respond in proportion.

Analysis by most of those concerned suggests that the difficulty lies not so much in the objective conditions, which are certainly not new, as in a public state of mind which demands improvement on many fronts at a rate faster than limited resources will allow. Most workers argue that these concerns bode well for the future of U.S. society. They are the mainsprings of action and social progress. Nevertheless, a general mood of criticism and contention prevails, and this is as true in the arena of health care as in many other areas of U.S. society. In this atmosphere, research on the health care system is forging ahead.

Currently the health services industry is America's third-largest and, given present growth rates, promises to be its largest in the near future. It employs over 4 million persons, of whom roughly 1 million are employed as professionals or sub-professionals (Rice and Cooper, 1969). In 1950, outlays on health totalled some $13 billion, and it is estimated that for the year 1969, such expenditures totalled over $60 billion (Cooper, 1969). Expenditures on health were $84 *per capita* in 1950, but were approximately $294 per member of the population in 1969 (Cooper, 1969). Outlays on health as a percentage of GNP equalled 4% in 1950, and currently they constitute nearly 7% of our nation's aggregate gross production of goods and services (Cooper, 1969).

Until five to ten years ago, the bulk of the information and analysis on economic aspects of health care was derived from a long succession of national commissions and congressional hearings in which most of the testimony came from persons and groups not trained in economics. By now, in contrast, the field of medical economics is active and, much outstanding economic talent is devoted to it. However, the research is still quite scattered, knowledge is fragmented, there are many gaps and fundamental facts are in dispute. The research on the whole has been closely identified with immediate practical problems and perhaps has not yielded the depth of insight or breadth of perspective that might have flowed from more basic investigation. There is as yet no monumental great book on the economics of health in America; thus the field appears ripe for systematic review and syntheses, as well as for further research on detailed aspects.

PROBLEMS AND ISSUES
Current U.S. social problems involving health include: the public's concern for the enormous rise in the prices and costs of health services as compared to other goods and services in the economy; the apparent lack of effectiveness in the nation's health care delivery system as compared to those of other developed nations; the unequal distribution of the availability of health services among various subgroups of the population; and special problems involving recent social legislation—Medicare and Medicaid.

The rise in medical costs and prices experienced in recent years has been spectacular, e.g. from 1950 to 1967 the consumer price index of medical care rose by 86% (from 73·4 to 136·7), and the consumer price index for all items rose by only 38% (from 83·8 to 116·3) (Rice and Cooper, 1969). If, as some believe, existing prices are below market clearing ones, additional rises of medical prices are likely to result in the future. The costs of certain health service items are already at levels beyond the capacity of low-income and even medium-income consumers to afford, and the prospect of future increases in costs is cause for considerable apprehension, if not fear.

Yet, in spite of recent enormous outlays on health services and the rapid acceleration in the costs of providing them, there is reason to call the effectiveness of the nation's health care delivery system into question. Only modest improvements in age-adjusted mortality have occurred in America in the past several decades. In 1965 the United States ranked eighteenth in infant mortality, twenty-second in male life expectancy, and tenth in female life expectancy among the developed nations of the world (Knowles, 1969). Such comparisons suggest that rapidly expanding outlays on health services are not yielding commensurate returns to the health of those residing in the United States.

A related concern is the growing awareness that health services are not equally available to all groups in our society. A maldistribution of health services exists; the relative shortages of health services among low-income earners—those residing in the central core of many of our nation's cities and those living in rural areas—is well-known. Maldistribution constitutes another barrier to accessibility to health services in addition to the financial barrier imposed by the high costs of services. Overcrowding leads to a deterioration of the warmth with which care is delivered and is a matter of concern to many Americans.

Finally, efforts to alleviate or solve certain of America's health service delivery problems, have both accentuated some old problems and produced new ones as well. Recent amendments to the Social Security Act, Titles 18 and 19—Medicare and Medicaid respectively—are designed to increase the availability of health services to the aged and medically-indigent in the United States. In the fiscal year 1968, some $5·8 billion of federal dollars were spent on health services under the auspices of these programmes, as contrasted with $1·6 billion in 1966. By 1969, this figure had climbed to over $11 billion. This tremendous increase in the funds available for purchasing health services on the behalf of those groups assisted by these programmes, undoubtedly had a great deal to do with the rapid acceleration of prices occurring over that interval of time. Yet, the mechanisms by which these funds are distributed, predominantly involving reimbursing suppliers of health services at 'cost', do little to alter the distribution of services available or to encourage the efficiency with which health services are produced and delivered. Indeed, many argue that the volume of funds expended thus far falls short of the volume needed and that existing reimbursement schemes have the undesirable consequence of expanding an industry which is lacking in effectiveness, efficiency, and equity.

In view of the importance of the problems confronting the health services sector of the economy and the challenges their analysis presents, the number of U.S. economists who have undertaken research in the area is growing rapidly.

In December 1967, a special breakfast session was held for medical economists during the Annual American Economic Convention. Some twenty health economists attended. This year, on December 29th, over 120 scholars attended a similar session. These figures are by no means indicative of the number of U.S. economists who are interested in health services research. The number who are so interested is much larger. However, the growth in attendance at these meetings is indicative of the rapid growth of health economics as an area of research specialisation in America.

The sheer volume of study on the economics of health care in America precludes our surveying the whole field. We propose, therefore, to outline the principal areas of current study and to report on a few examples of what may be regarded as notable research completed or in progress since 1965.

HEALTH ECONOMICS RESEARCH IN THE UNITED STATES

However, before discussing current research, two recent surveys of the field should be mentioned. The first is a small book sponsored by the Ford Foundation and written by Professor Herbert E. Klarman (formerly of Johns Hopkins University and now of New York University) entitled *The Economics of Health* (Columbia University Press, 1964). This book is a concise review of knowledge of U.S. health economics as of five years ago and contains an excellent bibliography of 230 items. The second survey is a two-volume report of a conference on health services research held in Chicago in late 1965. The report includes sixteen papers by leading U.S. scholars in the field of health economics and was published in the *Milbank Memorial Fund Quarterly* (vol. XLIV, Nos. 2 and 4, July and October 1966).

In addition to these volumes, the papers and proceedings of three recent conferences on the economics of health services are, or soon will be, available in print. The first, held in 1962 at Ann Arbor, Michigan, brought U.S. medical economic researchers together for the first time. The papers and proceedings of that conference, entitled the *Economics of Health and Medical Care* (University of Michigan Press, 1964), are representative of the work completed up to that time. A second conference on the economics of health services was held in December 1968 in Baltimore. The papers and proceedings of that conference and some additional papers that became available shortly thereafter are published in a volume entitled *Empirical Studies in Health Economics* (Johns Hopkins Press, 1970) under the editorship of Professor Herbert Klarman. Finally, the most recent conference on the economics of health services was held at the University of Iowa in September 1969. Of the ten papers presented by leading health researchers, eight were published in a special March 1970 edition of *Inquiry* (a scholarly journal published by the American Blue Cross Association).

The volumes mentioned above provide excellent overviews of the kinds of health economics research that have been undertaken in the United States and contain useful bibliographies as well.

A REVIEW OF SELECTED STUDIES

Several specific studies or lines of inquiry will now be summarised briefly in the interests of providing a better understanding of some of the major trends and developments in health economics research in the United States. Selection of a few items from a vast body of material is difficult and possibly invidious. Unfortunately, space does not permit the presentation of a more adequate sample.

Collection of Basic Statistics

Some of the most important research in the United States is the collection of continuing basic statistics on the health service system. This work is done chiefly by the federal government in the Bureau of Labour Statistics, Public Health Service, and Social Security Administration. Among the leaders in the field are three distinguished ladies: Ida Merriam, Dorothy Rice and Barbara Cooper.

Tables 1–6 (Appendix) present a few of these statistics; they convey an idea of the kind of information becoming available and at the same time provide an overview of the U.S. health services system.

Health Manpower

A great deal of concern has been expressed in the United States concerning apparent shortages of health manpower (Jeffers *et al.*, 1970). Numerous studies have been undertaken in an effort to determine whether or not shortages of key health professionals exist and what is in store for the future. While physicians have received considerable attention in this connection, studies of other health professions have been conducted as well. Space only permits limited attention to the topic.

One study that has received considerable attention in America was completed recently by Rashi Fein, formerly of the Brookings Institution and now of Harvard University, entitled *The Doctor Shortage, An Economic Diagnosis* (1967). In his book Fein provides estimates of the demand for and supply of physicians' services in 1975 and 1980 and draws policy conclusions from these estimates. He measures physicians' services in terms of the number of patient visits to physicians, and projects future demand in terms of the number of visits consumers would be prepared to purchase at 1965 relative prices. His findings (p. 60) are summarised in Table 7 (Appendix) showing 'the impact of demographic and socio-economic changes in the demand for physician visits over the period 1967–1975'. He expects an increase in demand of 21·9–25·8% by 1975 and of 35–40% by 1980.

Fein believes these percentage increases represent a lower limit, and he suggests that they may be raised by non-measurable factors such as new medical discoveries, new standards of medical care, increased availability of services, etc.

He estimates that the supply of physicians will increase from 1965 to 1975 by 19%, assuming continuation of the substantial immigration of doctors into the United States that has occurred since World War II. Thus, he concludes that supply will not keep up with demand to 1975, and he predicts that the disparity will be worse in 1980 than in 1975. However, the expected increase in the number of physicians will be sufficient to keep pace with population growth and on that basis he argues that no actual deterioration of service is likely. But the number of physicians would not grow enough to meet the demand derived from rising income and other causes.

He then attempts to analyse physician productivity. He finds that there was substantial improvement in productivity between 1950 and 1965 because of antibiotic drugs, increasing use of auxiliary personnel, improved organisation of practice, etc. He suggests that improved productivity in the future could close the gap between supply and demand, but he has reservations about whether this improvement will occur unless there are adequate incentives or pressures in this direction. He concludes that the future situation will be tight but not catastrophic. He emphasises that there will be little incentive from spontaneous private enterprise to supply more and better service to rural and poverty areas without specific public policies for these purposes.

Economies of Scale in Hospitals and Physician Practices
Given the apparent shortage of health professionals, considerable research has been directed toward ways of discovering how existing health production units can become more efficient. Major emphasis has been focussed on hospitals and physician office practices. Mention will be made of the work of three authors who have investigated possible cost economies in the case of hospitals and of two others who have studied 'economies of scale' in physician practices.

Ralph Berry, and John Caree and Paul Feldstein published at roughly the same time in 1967, separate papers on the relation of hospital size to average cost. In both studies, efforts were made to eliminate, or measure separately, variables other than size or scale. Berry approached the problem by grouping hospitals according to services and facilities provided to eliminate 'product differentiation'. Then, measuring the relation between size and cost per patient-day for each group, he found what in his mind is overwhelming evidence of declining average costs as size increased.

Carr and Feldstein (1967), also using multiple regression techniques, found 'that cost per patient-day falls initially as size is increased because of the economies associated with the use of specialised personnel and equipment', but that cost 'probably rises at very large-size levels due to increased managerial problems of communication and control' (p. 45). The optimum point for all hospitals appeared to be at about 190 patients (average daily census).

They discovered that optimum size tends to be higher for hospitals with a wide range of services than for those with a more limited range.

Two studies of economies of scale in physician practices have yielded conflicting results. Donald Yett's (1967) study revealed that substantial cost savings are possible as physicians' practices grow in size. However, Richard Bailey's (1970) intensive study of a sample of internists in the San Francisco Bay area, provides less optimistic results.

Yett, applying multiple regression analysis to data provided by mailed questionnaires yielding information on expenses, patient visits, and other variables, found that marginal costs decline over a substantial range of output of annual patient visits. Bailey, working with a much smaller sample of physicians, found that larger-scale practices (as revealed by the number of physicians working together in the same practice) produce fewer patient visits per physician per year. Physicians tend to work fewer hours per year when involved in a 'group practice', and the number of patients seen per hour by group-practice physicians seems not to differ drastically from the number of patients seen per hour by solo practitioners. Bailey found that net revenues are higher per patient visit in group practices due to the presence and utilisation of X-rays, laboratory services, etc., which are more frequently associated with group practices than with solo practices. The real issue in Bailey's mind is whether the use of ancillary personnel and more equipment really increases the productivity of physicians or whether these merely permit physicians to assign more services per patient visit and thus increase net revenues.

Organisation of Medical Practices

Considerable interest has been focussed on the desirability of reorganising America's existing pattern of health care delivery. Again, interest is centred on hospitals and physicians.

An interesting study conducted by Kenneth D. Rogers, Mary Mally and Florence L. Marcus in 1968, describes one of the myriad of experimental projects currently being conducted in America and elsewhere relating to the organisation of medical practice.

In this study, the experiment consisted of establishing a general medical practice for 2,500 persons in a low-income, public-housing area of Pittsburgh. The special feature of the practice was that the services of the single physician were augmented by those of a psychiatric social worker, public health nurse, office nurse, laboratory technician, and secretary-receptionist. Each of these auxiliary persons (except the secretary-receptionist) performed functions which would ordinarily be reserved for a physician. Also, the team as a whole provided more preventive and health education services than would be common in private practice. Tables 9 and 10 (Appendix) describe the division of labour among the members of the team.

The conclusions from the study were:

(a) that patients readily accepted non-physician personnel for services ordinarily reserved for physicians;

(b) that auxiliary personnel made it possible to render services not ordinarily provided by physicians in private practice; and

(c) that the quality of care both technically and in terms of warm human relationships was probably higher than that ordinarily available.

Medicare and Other Financial Mechanisms

In 1967, Dr and Mrs Somers of Princeton University published a major book, *Medicare and the Hospitals*, analysing the impact of Medicare and evaluating the new programme in its first year of operation. The book is so rich in detail that we cannot possibly summarise it all, so we shall mention only certain major conclusions about the impact of the Medicare system.

(1) Despite fears to the contrary, Medicare has not resulted in hospital crowding; and it appears that with good management, the hospital system is capable of handling the load for acute bed care. Medicare helps to relieve the hospitals by providing benefits for stays in extended-care facilities and for ambulatory care, and also by providing utilisation review in hospitals. However, out-patient facilities are inadequate, and there is need for their development. The U.S. system of autonomy of the physician, in relation to the hospital where he practices, will make this development difficult.

(2) The Somers believe that Medicare affects quality favourably. Standards of care are high; cost reimbursement is generous; segregation of patients by income, class and race is ended; and institutions to qualify for providing care must be certified. However, the effect on quality is expected to be a matter of grading up over time and is not a matter of instantaneous change.

(3) The personnel problems in U.S. hospitals are near the breaking

point. Medicare, which will increase patient load and raise standards of care, will increase the demand for personnel at all levels and accentuate the shortages. At the same time, Medicare will provide resources from which higher wages and salaries can be paid.

(4) A blunder was made in Medicare legislation when it was provided that hospital-based physicians (mainly anaesthesiologists, radiologists, pathologists and psychiatrists) would be paid by separate bills rendered to patients rather than by salaries. The effect was to raise cost and to set back the possibility of organised practice of medicine within hospitals.

(5) The Medicare legislation provides that hospitals will be reimbursed for services on the basis of 'reasonable costs' and physicians on the basis of 'reasonable charges'. This system has resulted in uncertainty about the meaning of the word 'reasonable' and in practice has made reimbursement open-ended with little provision for cost control. This reimbursement system is a major factor in the recent escalation of medical costs. Various proposals are emerging for cost control that will be compatible with the free-enterprise philosophy of U.S. health care, but none of these proposals has yet received wide acceptance. Some of these proposals include: increasing co-insurance and deductibles; public utility regulation; state surveillance of rates; a 'target rate' plan which involves an incentive bonus; and a 'capitation' plan which involves payment of a flat amount per patient instead of payment according to bed-days of use. (Note: since the publication of the Somers' book, the open-ended system of reimbursement has been tightened up.)

(6) The Medicare legislation gives some slight encouragement to community-wide planning of hospital services. Dr and Mrs Somers believe the law (the Comprehensive Health Planning Act, P. L. 89-749) should be modified to require community-wide planning—especially with reference to capital investment. Mandatory planning is, of course, not fully consistent with hospital autonomy.

(7) On the problem of rising costs, the Somers conclude (p. 257): 'The fact is that we do not yet know how—within the prevailing organisational structure—to pay for health services effectively through a mass-underwriting programme.'

Cost-Benefit and Cost-Effectiveness Analysis in America
Over a third of the total outlays for health in the United States were

K

made for services rendered in hospitals, the bulk of which are voluntary and non-profit-seeking. Denied of the resource-allocation properties of the free play of competitive markets, U.S. health decision-makers have had to look for analytical means of making such decisions which were, at least in part, not dependent on market variables. Considerable interest has been expressed in cost-benefit and cost-effectiveness methodologies as tools assisting decision-makers in making resource-allocation decisions relating to health programmes.

Concerning cost-benefit analysis, the paper chosen for discussion here is one written by Professor Herbert Klarman in 1968 in collaboration with Messrs Francis and Rosenthal on 'Cost-Effectiveness Analysis Applied to the Treatment of Chronic Renal Disease'. The problem in this paper was to compare, by means of cost-effectiveness analysis, the treatment of chronic renal disease by: dialysis administered at a hospital, dialysis administered at home, and kidney transplantation. The problem was highly relevant in the United States since, at the time of writing, 6,000 persons whose lives could be appreciably extended died annually from renal failure.

Estimates were made of the life-years gained by patients under the three treatments, with adjustments for the better quality of life of those having kidney transplants as compared with these having dialysis. Estimates were also made of the lifetime costs discounted to the present for the three types of treatment. Conclusions were reached by comparing life-years gained and present value of expenditures. The results are shown in Table 8 (Appendix). The authors conclude that transplantation is the most efficient way to increase the life expectancy of people with chronic kidney disease.

Econometric Models

While econometric methodologies are being used with increasing frequency in medical economic research, few have attempted to build a 'large model' of the health services industry. However, in December 1968, Paul J. Feldstein and Sander Kelman, both of the University of Michigan, presented a paper on 'A Framework for an Econometric Model of the Medical Care Sector'. In this paper they outlined in considerable detail a plan to develop a model of the entire market for medical care services. The purpose of the model is to develop a framework into which data could be fitted to explain the inputs of factors, the quantities of products, the costs, and the prices for all parts of the health care system. This model would be used 'to forecast the effect of changes in variables resulting either from changes in government policy or from changes in the factors affecting supply or demand conditions' and 'to enable policy-makers to improve their decision-making' (p. 172). The model considers eighty variables, forty-seven of which are determined by the equations of the model (endogenous variables); the remainder are treated as variables that exert an influence on the system but whose values are determined elsewhere (exegenous variables).

CONCLUDING COMMENTS

While brief summaries of only some of the more recent and significant studies provided here are grossly inadequate as a survey of the field of U.S. health economics, they do provide an impression of some problems that are being investigated and the ways that they are being approached by U.S. health service researchers.

We conclude with some comments concerning a widely shared hope that the United States may be able to construct a system of social accounts comparable to its national income accounts. Many congressional leaders and national commissions have pointed to the need to define goals, appraise social progress, and assess the social consequences of new technology and new policy. Many scholars believe that we know too little about social progress except in the economic sphere and that we urgently need reliable indices of trends in the status of minority groups, education, crime and delinquency, income distribution, housing, physical environment and health. It is suggested that if we had such data we might face some chastening surprises regarding the much-vaunted U.S. social progress. Such information might have a profound effect on social policy in the United States.

A first effort to produce a comprehensive study of social progress was completed a year ago. The report of this study was published by the Department of Health, Education and Welfare under the title *Toward a Social Report* (U.S. Government Printing Office, January 1969). The principal author was a very capable economist, Mancur Olson.

This document contains an interesting section on health which is addressed to the question: 'Are we getting healthier?' In preparing this report, trends in the incidence of various diseases were studied, changes in life expectancy recorded, and an interesting new indicator —'expectancy of a healthy life'—was developed covering the period since 1958. This indicator measures 'life expectancy free of bed disability and institutionalisation'. It takes account of all changes, good and bad, in either the amount of major disability or the level of death rates, yielding one net indicator of health. The weaknesses of the indicator are that it does not measure changes in amount of illness not involving bed disability, and it ignores progress in the reduction of discomfort and suffering. Nevertheless, it appears to be a useful indicator of social progress in the field of health (see Table 10, Appendix).

As shown in Table 10, health progress, as measured either by expectation of life or expectation of healthy life, has been less than dramatic in the past decade. This is in contrast to important advances, at least in life expectancy, over the years prior to 1958. So, America appears to be faced with the irony that at precisely the time when expenditures for health care and health research have been sky-rocketing, progress in health itself has been nearly at a standstill. This fact would not be disturbing if the United States was a world leader in the health of its people. The facts are, as the *Social Report* shows (pp. 6–7): 15 nations have a longer life expectancy at birth; 13 are ahead of the United States in infant mortality; 5 surpass us in maternal mortality; and we are far from the top in death rates from TB and pneumonia.

Health is, of course, a resultant of many factors, of which the health service system is only one. But the available evidence is not reassuring about the U.S. health care system.

One final comment. Virtually every known study in the field of health economics refers to lack of adequate knowledge and the need for additional research. While there is great need for the gathering of more reliable data and the generation of new ideas, there are many facets of the health care field that will not yield to research in the sense of objective and quantifiable facts and relationships. With all conceivable empirical knowledge, there will be great need for wisdom, judgement, intuition and sensitivity to moral values in reaching sound practical decisions. It is gratifying that in America the field of medical economics is active in attracting outstanding economic talent, but it also needs statesmen and philosophers as well as economists.

REFERENCES

Bailey, R., 'Philosophy, Faith and Facts (?) in the Production Medical Services', *Inquiry*, March 1970.

Berry, R. E., 'Returns to Scale in the Production of Hospital Services', *Health Services Research*, Summer 1967.

Carr, J. W., and Feldstein, P. J., 'The Relationship of Cost to Hospital Size', *Inquiry*, June 1967.

Cooper, Barbara S., 'National Health Expenditures, Fiscal Years 1929–69, and Calendar Years 1929–1968', *Research and Statistics, Note: Social Security Administration*, November 7, 1969.

Fein, R., *The Doctor Shortage: An Economic Diagnosis*, The Brookings Institution, Washington D.C. 1967.

Feldstein, P. J., and Kelman, S., 'A Framework for an Econometric Model of the Medical Care Sector', in: Klarman, H. E. (ed.), *Empirical Studies in Health Economics*, Baltimore 1970 (The Johns Hopkins Press).

Jeffers, J. R., Bognanno, M., and Bartlett, J. C., 'On the Demand vs. Need for Medical Services and the Concept of Shortage', *American Journal of Public Health*, 1970.

Klarman, H. E., Francis, J. O's., and Rosenthal, G. D., 'Cost Effectiveness Analysis Applied to the Treatment of Chronic Renal Disease', *Medical Care*, January-February 1968.

Knowles, J. H., 'The Quantity and Quality of Medical Manpower: A Review of Medicine's Current Efforts', *Journal of Medical Education*, February 1969.

Rice, Dorothy P., and Cooper, Barbara D., 'National Health Expenditures, 1950–67', *Social Security Bulletin*, January 1969.

Rogers, K. D., Mally, Mary, and Marcus, Florence L., 'A General Medical Practice Using Non-Physician Personnel', *Journal of the American Medical Association*, November 1968.

Somers, H., and Somers, Anne R., *Medicare and the Hospitals*, The Brookings Institution, Washington D.C. 1967.

Yett, D. E., 'An Evaluation of Alternative Methods of Estimating Physicians Expenses Relative to Output', *Inquiry*, March 1967.

APPENDICES

Table 1. Expenditures for Health Services by Type of Expenditure and Source of Funds, 1967 ($ millions)

| Type of Expenditure | Total | Source of Funds | | | | | | |
| | | Private | | | | Public | | |
		Total	Con-sumers	Philan-thropy	Other	Total	Federal	State and Local
Professional services								
Physicians	10,163	8,201	8,191	10	–	1,962	1,375	587
Dentists	3,186	3,063	3,063	–	–	124	68	55
Other	1,447	1,348	1,323	25	–	98	60	39
Sub-total	14,796	12,612	12,577	35	–	2,184	1,503	681
Manufactured products								
Drugs and drug sundries	5,569	5,337	5,337	–	–	232	120	112
Eyeglasses and appliances	1,584	1,545	1,545	–	–	39	19	20
Sub-total	7,153	6,882	6,882	–	–	271	139	132
Institutional care								
Hospitals	17,946	9,092	8,752	340	–	8,854	5,549	3,306
Nursing homes	1,858	666	646	20	–	1,192	775	418
Sub-total	19,804	9,758	9,398	360	–	10,046	6,324	3,724
Expenses for pre-payment and administration	1,777	1,560	1,560	–	–	217	217	–
Government public health activities	914	–	–	–	–	914	268	646
Research	1,775	178	–	178	–	1,597	1,530	67
Construction	1,995	1,158	–	579	579	837	432	405
Other	2,441	685	–	315	370	1,856	1,412	344
Grand total	50,655	32,833	30,417	1,467	949	17,822	11,825	5,999

Source: Dorothy P. Rice and Barbara D. Cooper, 'National Health Expenditures, 1950–1967', *Social Security Bulletin*, January 1969, p. 4.

Table 2. Expenditures for Health Services, 1950–1967 ($ millions)

	1950	1955	1960	1965	1966	1967
Professional services						
Physicians	2,755	3,680	5,684	8,745	9,156	10,163
Dentists	975	1,525	1,977	2,808	2,964	3,186
Other	395	559	862	1,038	1,258	1,447
Sub-total	4,125	5,764	8,523	12,591	13,378	14,796
Manufactured products						
Drug & drug sundries	1,730	2,385	3,657	4,850	5,217	5,569
Eyeglasses & appliances	490	597	776	1,230	1,406	1,584
Sub-total	2,220	2,982	4,433	6,080	6,623	7,153
Institutional care						
Hospitals	3,845	5,429	9,044	13,520	15,414	17,946
Nursing homes	142	222	526	1,328	1,526	1,852
Sub-total	3,987	6,151	9,570	14,848	16,940	19,804
Expenses for pre-payment & administration	300	614	863	1,297	1,628	1,777
Government public health activities	361	377	412	696	778	914
Research	117	216	662	1,469	1,623	1,775
Construction	840	721	1,048	1,912	1,955	1,995
Other	917	1,211	1,462	1,698	2,081	2,441
Grand total	12,867	18,036	26,973	40,591	45,006	50,655

Source: Rice and Cooper, *op. cit.*, p. 12.

Table 3. Indexes of Medical Care Prices Compared with the Consumer Price Index (1957–60 = 100)

Year	Consumer Price Index: All Items	Medical Care Total	Physician Fees	Dentist Fees	Optometric Exam. & Eyeglasses	Hospital Daily Service Charges	Prescriptions & Drugs
1940	48·8	50·3	54·5	53·5	70·8	25·4	69·3
1945	62·7	57·5	63·3	63·3	77·8	32·5	73·2
1950	83·8	73·4	76·0	81·5	89·5	57·8	86·6
1955	93·3	88·6	90·0	93·1	93·8	83·0	92·7
1960	103·1	108·1	106·0	104·7	103·7	112·7	102·3
1965	109·9	122·3	121·5	117·6	113·0	153·3	98·1
1966	113·1	127·7	128·5	121·4	116·1	168·0	98·4
1967	116·3	136·7	137·6	127·5	121·8	200·1	97·9
1968	121·2	145·0	145·3	134·5	125·7	226·6	98·1
1968 (Dec.)	123·7	149·1	149·1	137·3	127·6	239·3	98·5
1969 (June)	127·6	155·2	155·5	144·2	131·2	253·8	99·3

Source: Bureau of Labor Statistics, Consumer Price Index.

Table 4. Health Services Manpower and Facilities

	1950	1955	1960	1965	1966
Physicians, M.D. + D.O.	232,697	255,211	274,834	305,115	313,559
per 100,000 population	149	150	148	153	156
Physicians, in private practice*	168,000	169,900	179,200	190,800	
per 100,000 civilian population	109	102	98	97	98
Dentists	87,164	94,879	101,947	109,301	111,622
per 100,000 population	57	57	56	56	56
Dentists, active non-federal	75,313	76,087	82,630	86,317	88,025
per 100,000 population	50	47	46	45	45
Nurses, active prof. grad.	375,000	430,000	504,000	621,000	550,000
per 100,000 population	249	259	282	319	298
Hospital personnel, full-time equiv.	1,058,000	1,301,000	1,598,000	1,952,000	2,106,000
per 100 patients	84	95	114	139	151
Hospital beds, non-federal					
Short-term	504,504	567,612	639,057	741,292	768,479
per 100,000 population	334	348	359	386	396
Other	951,321	1,036,796	1,018,913	962,230	910,179
per 100,000 population	964	984	931	887	865
Total	1,455,825	1,604,408	1,657,970	1,703,522	1,678,658

* Prior to 1965 includes only physicians in private practice; also, in 1966, includes physicians rendering patient care in institutional settings.
Source: Statistical Abstract of the United States, 1966, pp. 65, 75, 76; 1967, p. 66; 1968, pp. 66, 67–70.

Table 5. Finance of Health Care Expenditures, 1950–1967 ($ millions)

	1950	1955	1960	1965	1966	1967	Increase: 1967 over 1950
Total expenditures	12,867	18,036	26,973	40,591	45,006	50,655	37,788
Less: Expenditures for purposes other than formal health care*	1,758	2,103	3,215	5,649	6,264	6,776	5,018
Expenditures for personal health care	11,109	15,933	23,758	34,942	38,742	43,879	32,770
Out-of-pocket expenditures	7,209	9,271	13,068	18,171	19,407	19,312	12,103
Third-party payments	3,900	6,662	10,690	16,771	19,335	24,567	20,667
Private health insurance	992	2,536	4,996	8,729	9,142	9,545	8,553
Government	2,588	3,705	5,157	7,345	9,449	14,257	11,669
Philanthropy and other	320	421	537	697	744	765	445

* Includes expenses for pre-payment and administration, government public health activities, and expenditures of private voluntary agencies in other health services.
Source: Rice and Cooper, *op. cit.,* p. 16.

Table 6. Geographic Disparities in Health Care Facilities, 1966 (rates per 100,000 population)

State	Physicians in Private Practice*	Active Dentists	Active Nurses (Professional graduate)**	Hospital Beds (Short-term)
New York	136	67	388	444
California	134	50	324	352
Colorado	126	53	370	432
Massachusetts	122	58	502	447
Connecticut	121	57	440	325
North Carolina	71	27	231	350
South Dakota	73	39	270	470
Arkansas	68	28	120	335
South Carolina	64	20	214	325
Alaska	65	26	287	218
Mississippi	60	25	142	322

* Included physicians rendering patient care in institutional settings.
** Data for 1962. Later figures not available.
Source: Statistical Abstract of the United States, 1968, p. 67.

Table 7. Estimated Percentage Increases in Demand for Physician Visits Deriving from Various Demographic and Socio-Economic Changes, 1965–1975

Change	Resulting Percentage Increase in Physician Visits
Population Growth	12·2 – 14·6
Age–sex distribution	1·0 – 1·0
Migration	0·2 – 0·2
Race	0·5 – 0·5
Education and income	7·0 – 7·5
Medicare	1·0 – 2·0
Total	21·9 – 25·8

Source: R. Fein, *The Doctor Shortage*, Brookings Institution, Washington D.C. 1967, p. 60.

Table 8. Estimated Present Value of Expenditures and Life-Years gained from Various Treatments of Chronic Renal Disease

	Present Value of Expenditures ($)	Life-Years Gained	Cost per Life-Year ($)
Hospital dialysis	104,000	9	11,600
Home dialysis	38,000	9	4,200
Transplantation (unadjusted)*	44,500	17	2,600
Transplantation (adjusted for quality of life)*	44,500	20·5	2,200

* Cost of transplantation includes $24,500 for dialysis for cases who return to dialysis after failure of transplant.
Source: H. E. Klarman, J. O'S. Francis and G. D. Rosenthal, 'Cost-Effectiveness Analysis Applied to the Treatment of Chronic Renal Disease', *Medical Care*, January–February 1968, p. 53.

Table 9. Percentage of Chief Health Problems Managed by Various Staff Members

Health Problem	Total (No.)	Physi- cian (%)	Technician Assistant (%)	Social Worker (%)	Office Nurse (%)	Visiting Nurse (%)
Psychological	862	24	–	73	2	1
Blood	213	84	2	–	13	–
Respiratory	2,007	72	1	–	23	4
Eye and ear	355	69	1	–	23	7
Digestive	436	73	2	–	14	10
Neurological	147	52	–	–	4	43
Genitourinary	239	59	1	–	5	35
Musculoskeletal	499	56	2	–	15	27
Cardiovascular	770	43	9	–	13	34
Endocrine	354	33	8	–	9	50
Skin	883	40	15	–	39	6
Whole-body*	856	40	11	–	30	11
Not ill**	450	67	12	–	17	4
Total	8,071	55	5	8	19	13

* Whole-body disease included acute febrile systemic disease of unknown etiology and nutritional disorders.
** Not ill included visits for well-baby, prenatal, and post-partum care, as for immunisation and periodic health appraisal.
Source: K. D. Rogers, Mary Mally and Florence L. Marcus, 'A General Medical Practice Using Nonphysician Personnel', *Journal of the American Medical Association*, November 18, 1968, p. 1,755.

Table 10. Percentage of Total Service in Each Category Given by Specific Staff Members

Service Category	Total (No.)	Physi- cian (%)	Technician Assistant (%)	Social Worker (%)	Office Nurse (%)	Visiting Nurse (%)
Physical examina- tion, complete	611	100	–	–	–	–
Physical examina- tion, partial	5,437	61	4	–	22	13
Counselling and education	2,186	18	3	23	17	39
Dressing—treat- ment	947	23	18	–	36	23
Laboratory tests	1,033	–	76	–	23	–
Screening tests and immunisa- tion	167	31	36	–	32	–
Medication dis- pensed/pre- scribed	4,527	96	1	–	1	2
Other (includes bedside nursing)	263	5	–	46	5	43
Total	15,171	59	9	4	15	13

Source: Rogers, Mally and Marcus, *loc. cit.*

Table 11. Expectation of Healthy Life, 1958–1966 (years)

Year	Expectation of Life	Expected Bed-Disability and Institutionalisation during Life	Expectation of Healthy Life
At Birth			
1958	69·5	2·3	67·2
1959	69·6	1·8	67·8
1960	69·9	2·0	67·9
1961	69·9	1·9	68·0
1962	70·2	2·1	68·1
1963	70·0	2·1	67·9
1964	69·9	2·0	67·9
1965	70·2	2·0	68·2
1966	70·2	2·0	68·2
At Age 65			
1958	14·2	1·1	13·1
1959	14·3	1·0	13·3
1960	14·5	1·1	13·4
1961	14·4	1·1	13·3
1962	14·6	1·1	13·5
1963	14·4	1·1	13·3
1964	14·3	1·1	13·2
1965	14·6	1·1	13·5
1966	14·6	1·1	13·5

Source: U.S. Department of Health, Education and Welfare, *Toward a Social Report*, Washington D.C., January 1969, pp. 3–4 (U.S. Government Printing Office).

Chapter VII

SUMMARY OF MAIN POINTS RAISED IN DISCUSSION

SUMMARY OF MAIN POINTS RAISED IN DISCUSSION

M. M. HAUSER

Institute of Social and Economic Research University of York

INTRODUCTION

The following points about the scope of the summary of the discussion should be emphasised at the outset. First, the proponents of particular contributions to the discussion are not identified by name. Second, no attempt has been made to include every statement made by contributors. Third, it is worth emphasising that no conscious effort was made at the conference to arrive at a consensus view on particular issues. Hence when we say, for example, that there was 'wide agreement' among participants on a particular point, this statement should be seen as reflecting the rapporteur's personal assessment of the discussion.

CONCEPTUAL PROBLEMS

Objective Targets

On various occasions during the conference participants touched, either directly or indirectly, upon what is commonly referred to by economists as the 'objective function' of medical care systems. Any attempt to understand and assess the operation of a medical care system, either in whole or in part, must begin by identifying the objective targets to be achieved by the system. For example, at the highest level it might be said that the main objective of medical care is to maximise the health of the community for a given input of resources. Or, again, it might be argued that the goal is to provide a comprehensive system of health services for all who are in need of them at some predetermined level. But clearly, specifications of this kind are not specific enough for assessment and planning purposes. In the last analysis, what is required is the formulation of a set of detailed objectives for individual services. The problem of defining these objectives, while recognised by participants as fundamental to the discussion and assessment of the role of medical care, was, however, not explored in detail at the conference.

In a democratic society the specification of targets is closely bound up with the central problem of revealing preferences. In theory, as is well-known, there are two distinct approaches to this problem: in a market-oriented system the revelation of preferences is achieved essentially by way of a pricing mechanism, while in a non-market context, like that prevailing in the British health services structure today, the solution is effected by other means, viz. by the substitution of a political process for the operation of the market place. There was frequent mention, but very little specific discussion, of this dichotomy at the conference. However, on a more general level, several participants expressed serious reservations about the practical applicability of the traditional doctrine of consumer sovereignty to the area of health care. What role can be assigned to consumer valuation in this area? The doctrine of consumer sovereignty rests on the assumptions of perfect market knowledge and rational behaviour by consumers. The question that arises here is: how far are these conditions (and especially the one concerning full market knowledge) satisfied in the case of medical care? Clearly, as one participant intimated, the answer to this question is important, because if in the last analysis it is decided that consumer valuations are irrelevant, then we need not waste time and effort devising methods of revealing consumer preferences and gauging consumer satisfaction.

There was divided opinion on the answer to this question, but this division was more one of degree than of principle. On the one hand, some conferees felt inclined to argue that medical care was in fact an area where there might be some justification for departing from the principle of strict consumer sovereignty. Medical care, it was said, is an area where, due to the highly technical and complex nature of medicine and lack of relevant information, consumers are frequently simply not competent to make intelligent judgements about some of the choices open to them. Hence it is an area where the traditional model of consumer sovereignty can be applied at best only to a limited degree. Of course, the question which then arises is: who should decide in place of the consumer? Should it be the producers (doctors), the politicians or perhaps the central administrators? One conferee argued strongly in favour of the doctor: the best defence of the consumer in medical care rests with the technically-qualified expert, even if admittedly the knowledge of the latter is limited.

On the other hand, other participants felt inclined to insist more emphatically on the potential role and importance of consumer valuation and choice. It was argued that there is clearly much more to medical care than merely technical factors, and in this sense there are also many conceivable areas where direct consumer choice might be expected to play a decisive role. Numerous examples can be cited to illustrate this point (availability of medical care, choice of doctor, choice of hospital and type of accommodation desired, etc.). If it is true that the information for consumers is lacking in many respects, there might be some gain in making efforts to improve the situation. Conversely, if there are areas where consumers are demonstrably incapable or incompetent of making rational judgements, it might be appropriate to clearly specify and single out the areas in question more clearly.

The uncertainty surrounding the potential importance of consumer preferences and choice in medical care was clearly highlighted at one particular point in the debate when a participant, in the course of a discussion of the potential role of screening, put the following question to the conference for consideration. Suppose it is known that there is a definite public demand for a particular screening programme—i.e. in a market system people would be prepared to pay a (money) price for the supply of the service—but assume also that, in the estimation of the central decision-makers responsible for the provision of the service, the latter is held to be ineffective—i.e. to have no technical payoff. Would those deciding on its provision in a system like the NHS be justified in denying the supply of the service to the public, on the ground that in their estimation the service is held to be of no value?

The conference showed division over the precise answer to this proposition. Two conferees thought that when formulated in this simplified manner, the question revealed a situation which was highly hypothetical and which could not be answered *a priori* with a simple yes or no. The decision to provide or not to provide a screening service will depend on a number of factors besides consumer demand, above all on the amount of resources that would be required to grant the service. Depending on whether or not the commitment of resources would need to be heavy, the decision might well vary.

A number of participants were inclined to take a more uncompromising view and maintained essentially that screening which showed no payoff should not be provided. As one conferee put it: where scientific investigation clearly shows that a service is ineffective the central administrators might be right in denying the provision of the service. Another conferee referred to the case where a disease is known to be incurable. In such a case it might be appropriate to resist consumer demand for screening, especially if the resources required to provide the screening service can be employed more effectively elsewhere in the system.

Against this, other participants felt inclined to argue that, given the conditions specified in the question, something would probably have to be done by the central administrators to meet public demand. The view that screening should be provided only if in the eyes of the experts it promises to show a payoff, is perhaps too narrow. One participant referred to the United States where, apparently, screening services are provided frequently regardless of whether or not there is a (technical) payoff attached to them. The crucial question is: what is one trying to maximise in medical care? Is it economic or technical payoff in a narrow sense or is it some sort of welfare measured by some appropriate index of health? In a sense, the case of screening might be compared with the case of the provision of placebos. These are known to be intrinsically ineffective substances but they nevertheless have a moral and suggestive effect on patients. They reduce their anxieties and provide them with reassurance. These are perfectly legitimate objectives of any medical care system and, although not always reflected in tangible economic gain, perhaps also ground enough for allowing the provision of a particular screening service.

Production Functions, Technical and Economic Efficiency

In connection with the discussion of objective targets for medical care and their achievement, the conference also turned its attention briefly to the notion of the 'production function' for medical care and, allied to this, to the distinction between technical and economic efficiency in the delivery of health care.

From the medical point of view, it can be said that the first aim of any medical care system is to reduce or prevent disease in the best possible manner, i.e. to bring to patients the maximum benefit in solving or ameliorating their clinical problems, given a certain state of medical knowledge at a particular point in time. In terms of standard economic theory the task here is essentially a medical question, involving what is commonly referred to as the *technical or productive efficiency* of different forms of treatment of disease, and aiming ultimately at formulating suitable *production functions* for the delivery of medical care, i.e. technical relations setting out the quantitative relationships between different sets of factor inputs and the corresponding (maximum) 'product' outputs, within the limitations set by a given state of medical knowledge at a particular point in time.

Economists are, on the whole, not particularly concerned with this problem of maximising a physical measure of output under given conditions regarding factor inputs and technical relationships. Their aim extends beyond the production function and technical efficiency as such and centres on another type of efficiency, namely *economic efficiency*. To this end economists tend to reason from a standpoint in which there exist a number of technically efficient processes for the achievement of a particular result and then proceed, by way of the introduction of a budget constraint and factor prices, to select that process which is economically best (cheapest) in achieving the desired result. In this sense it can be said that economists are concerned with value relationships (economic efficiency) rather than volume relationships (technical efficiency).

Several participants registered doubts about certain aspects of this approach as applied to medical care, especially about the prospect of formulating suitable production functions for different types of treatment. One conferee urged economists to turn away from the conventional idea of the production function in the case of health care and explore alternative possibilities of analysis. He thought that the conventional notion of the detailed production function is of questionable operational value in this area (as, indeed, it frequently is, even in industry!). Another participant suspected that in a great number of cases the production functions in medical care would turn out to be unique (i.e. there would not be different ways to achieve identical results). In cases of this kind the question of choice between processes according to economic criteria becomes meaningless. Several conferees made allusion to the fact that medical science quite often knows very little precisely about the quantitative (and, indeed, qualitative!) effects of different forms of treatment. The fact which must be faced is that in medical science as in other sciences, the greater part of knowledge is uncertain and speculative. As a result, the setting up of clearly defined production functions in the above sense becomes questionable, and the assumptions made by economists of given technical relationships simply cannot be upheld. Moreover, frequently new methods and processes are devised which subsequently never reach fruition, either because they are proved technically worthless or because they are overtaken by progress before they have been fully assessed, even in a medical sense. In cases of this kind the stage of economic assessment in the above sense is never even reached. Again, on some occasions a full medical and economic assessment may be largely irrelevant because public pressure makes it imperative to introduce a new method of treatment, irrespective of a comprehensive assessment of all its possible outcomes.

One participant thought that medical scientists would find it difficult to adopt the economist's approach and think in terms of a choice between technically efficient processes according to economic considerations. The choice problem confronting medical decision-makers is different: it is essentially to select among different forms of treatment that particular form which promises the greatest chance of success in improving the health of a patient. A choice in terms of economic costs and benefits does not enter directly into this.

Against these various reservations and in defence of the traditional approach there seemed, nevertheless, to be some agreement that the conventional notion of the production function and the distinction between technical and economic efficiency *could* serve a useful purpose in the analysis of medical care, if only to serve as a guide to practical assessment by focussing attention on the basic choices which have to be made, both technically in terms of factor substitution and economically in terms of opportunity costs and scarce resources. The problems in medical care (as, indeed, in other areas of economic activity) cannot be seen in terms of unconstrained maximisations. Admittedly, conventional notions are seldom encountered in pure form in practice, but at the same time in practice the problem is seldom to formulate an ideal solution; it is rather to attain a feasible result capable of improving a given situation.

'Shortages' in Medical Care Provision

Another topic which gave rise to some spirited discussion at the conference was the concept of 'shortage' in the provision of medical care.

There was no consensus view on the meaning of this concept among the participants. Non-economists frequently interpret the concept rather loosely: if more resources were available, then more and better medical care could be provided. There was, however, wide agreement that this particular notion of 'shortage' is too imprecise to be useful operationally. A more restricted and meaningful interpretation can be attained by relating the idea of 'shortage' to the notion of some accepted target levels of output. A 'shortage' of medical care provision can then be said to exist as long as the accepted target level of output is not achieved. For example, in this sense it might be said that there is a 'shortage' of doctors if there are not enough physicians to perform a prescribed number of operations.

Economists see the concept of 'shortage' predominantly in the context of a relationship between quantity and price. A 'shortage' of provision indicates that the prevailing price for the commodity in question is too low. Several participants underlined the importance of this particular notion of 'shortage' for the optimal allocation of resources, not merely at the level of the economy as a whole between alternative objectives, but also in a more limited sense within the medical care system itself. 'Shortages' in a technical sense, it was said, occur all the time and everywhere. This is not the main problem facing the decision-maker. The central (economic) problem lies in the fact that available resources are limited, and that in order to achieve an efficient allocation of these resources one should be able to judge the relative importance of the various ends toward which these resources can be employed, i.e. one should be able to evaluate the magnitude of the shortages which occur in different directions and weigh them against each other. This calls for two distinct but related steps, namely: first, for the establishment of a workable mechanism to evaluate the magnitude of the various shortages; and second, for the identification of a common yardstick to enable a comparison to be made between the relative value to be attached to reducing each of the various shortages (the estimation of trade-offs). In a democratic society the first step is effected either by a market mechanism or, in the absence of a market mechanism, by politicians. In respect to the second step, the obvious yardstick which suggests itself, at least to economists, is money, though the evaluations of politicians are seldom cast (explicitly at least) in these terms.

One participant said that despite the above-mentioned mechanisms for making choices, the plain fact is that there is at present no satisfactory method in practice of arriving at scientific assessments of priorities and rational evaluations of trade-offs between different resource uses, either at the macro-economic level or within the more restricted area of the medical care system itself. The first difficulty which arises in the case of medical care in this context is that economists and non-economists (doctors) tend to have different views about output. Medical scientists see output predominantly in medical/humanitarian terms, whereas economists have tended to see output predominantly in economic terms, and are inclined to want to attach money prices to the values under consideration. A second difficulty rests in the fact that comparisons between people always involve subjective judgements. Other problems are of a more directly practical nature, e.g. the confusion which can at times be observed in respect of the notion of costs in an accounting sense (cash movements) and in an economic sense (foregone opportunities).

One participant qualified the request for a formalisation of all benefits and trade-offs in terms of a common yardstick. Insofar as the weighing-up process is done by persons individually, he said, there is no need for an objective formalisation. The individual will employ his own yardstick. Other conferees expressed doubts about the practicability of expressing all relevant values in terms of a single measure. For some values in the area of health care, it was observed, expression in terms of a uni-dimensional measure is extremely difficult, if not impossible. The problem of evaluating such magnitudes as the saving of human life and the physical and psychic benefits resulting from reduced suffering and anxiety, both to the individual and to his family, could be mentioned as illustrations in this context.

Against this, other participants insisted on the need to express all values in terms of a common yardstick. The specification of such a measure is essential to a proper and objective comparison between different trade-offs. The addition of humanitarian benefits to the array of values changes nothing in principle. The fact is that there are always trade-offs between different potential resource uses, whatever the intrinsic nature of these trade-offs may be. In the last analysis all values, including humanitarian values, should be expressed in terms of the accepted common yardstick.

A short exchange of views also developed on the role played by the economist in the above valuation process. Some economists, it was alleged, tend to think predominantly in terms of economic efficiency. However, even they had to admit that there are other objectives in medical care besides economic efficiency. In this sense it is clear that economists have a part to play in the assessment of medical care, but the final decisions as well as the weighting of various trade-offs between objectives, cannot rest with them but must be determined by other people, namely the politicians. Partly in elaboration of this point and partly in reply to it, other participants, while not denying the role played by the politicians, thought nevertheless that in the present circumstances economists had a vital role to play in assisting in the decision-making process relating to the health care system. By analysing the economic implications of alternative projects and ranking the latter according to their economic viability, the economist can contribute vitally to the formulation of proper solutions to some of the central problems facing the medical care system today.

Need and Demand

The question of the difference between the two distinct but related concepts of 'need' and 'demand' for medical care was another significant topic discussed at some length at the conference.

Some participants tried to give appropriate definitions for the two concepts of 'need' and 'demand' for medical care. In a general sense it could be argued that a 'need' for medical care will exist whenever an individual is in a position where he could benefit from the application of health care. However, this says nothing about in whose judgement the individual is likely to benefit. In principle, the judgement could be made by any one of a number of conceivable agents, e.g. by the individual himself, by the medical experts (doctors), by the politicians, by the central decision-makers of a particular programme according to what they interpret to be in the consumers' best interest, or, in an even wider sense, by the community as a whole.

The concept of 'demand' is more specific and narrower in scope than 'need'. According to standard economic theory, 'demand' implies the notion of a resource sacrifice in exchange for the acquisition of a commodity or service, i.e. the willingness on the part of the purchaser to pay a price for the satisfaction of an individual need. In this sense 'demand' can be regarded as that part of individual 'need' which is transformed into a definite and concrete request for services by the patient. The question here is how far the individual is able to meet his need.

One participant registered some concern over the attempt to give generally valid definitions for the concepts of 'need' and 'demand' for medical care. In his view these are terms which cannot be defined in a unified manner once for all, since they are likely to be employed and interpreted differently in different contexts and disciplines relating to the health service structure. Other conferees questioned the usefulness of the distinction between 'need' and 'demand'. One participant had doubts especially about the usefulness of the concept of 'need' and expressed the view that of the two concepts of 'need' and 'demand', only the latter could be regarded as (operationally) useful. Another participant questioned even the usefulness of 'demand'. 'Demand', so his argument went, is essentially a functional relationship between quantity and price and hence operationally less useful than consumption, for example, which at any one time is an objective and observable fact.

Other participants took a contrasting view and maintained that the distinction between 'need' and 'demand' was relevant. The two concepts are in some ways related, but clearly distinct and useful. The 'demand' and 'need' of an individual may coincide; but alternatively there may also be a definite 'need' but no 'demand'. For example, in cases where income is deficient or where individuals are unable to decide for themselves or where externalities are involved, there may be a definite 'need' for a particular individual to consume a particular medical service, but personally the individual may not be in a position or may not choose to exercise a demand for that service. Again, there may be a 'need' for a particular service, but for some reason or other that 'need' is not allowed to express itself in 'demand' (e.g. abortions).

In one of the conference papers the notion of 'demand' was described as follows: '*Demand* (active, effective) for public care is that part of the need for care which is represented by those individuals who come in touch with the system of public care with a desire for consultation and treatment, and who are willing to wait if this cannot be provided at once. In each period demand takes the form of queueing or results in *consumption* (i.e. satisfied demand)' (J.-E. Spek, p.

265). One participant, in making allusion to this particular definition, wondered how far it was legitimate to include in a definition of 'demand' a statement to the effect that individuals must be 'willing to wait' (queue) if consultation and treatment cannot be provided at once. Some conferees replied that in a situation like that prevailing today in Britain, Sweden and other countries, 'waiting' (queueing) had clearly become a significant element in the demand for medical care. As said earlier, 'demand' implies on the part of the consumer a willingness to sacrifice resources for the acquisition of medical care, i.e. within his budget constraint to pay a price for this purpose. Depending on the conditions facing individual consumers this price may take the form of money or, alternatively, time. In a sense, 'waiting' is hence equivalent to 'paying' in terms of money, and in many cases money and time can be traded against each other. This question of paying in terms of time could be of particular importance in a non-market situation, it was said, because it touches clearly upon the question of how resources are allocated and hence provides a certain alternative to a regular market mechanism.

There was very little discussion about the assumptions and implications inherent in this approach, although some participants were clearly critical about the assumption of viewing the size of 'waiting-lists' and 'queues' as measures of demand. The concept of a queue, it was argued, is a complex phenomenon, e.g. a queue at a university medical care institution is something entirely different from a queue at a private practice. The meaning and importance of a waiting-list in a particular case is difficult to interpret and its relationship to demand is by no means simple.

PROBLEMS OF ECONOMIC ASSESSMENT

Social Accounting and Medical Care

The application of social accounting methods to the analysis of the health care system (as undertaken in one of the conference papers) was welcomed by a number of participants as a promising and pioneering development in the economic appraisal of medical care. A description of the system in this form, it was stated, can serve a useful purpose in improving the overall understanding of this system, and also in facilitating the assessment of eventual changes in this system.

One conferee observed that an equivalent approach exists at present only for one other area of economic activity, namely education.

Another participant expressed the view that while the framework would undoubtedly prove useful to the work of the economist in health care, it would presumably be of little or no relevance to the work of the medical profession. Other members, while generally in favour of the idea, advised caution in the further exploration of the approach in relation to medical care. It is a well-known fact, it was said, that the traditional social accounting framework is in several respects severely limited; hence it cannot be assumed that the method is amenable to every conceivable purpose. Its suitability for purposes of economic assessment needs to be carefully reviewed from case to case and, if necessary, adapted and expanded to meet particular conditions.

Several members pointed out some of the shortcomings and problems inherent in endeavouring to apply social accounting methods to the health care system. The following summary provides a brief outline of some of the more prominent points which were raised in this context.

(1) In the last analysis, in medical care as in many other areas, one is not concerned in the first place with output in national income terms, but with *welfare* (all goods and values which have utility for people). Output in the national income sense, as employed in social accounting, can serve at best as a proxy for welfare.

(2) The present social accounting framework is essentially static— it incorporates no dynamic elements.

(3) In Britain the evaluation of output in health presents serious difficulties, owing to the fact that for wide areas of the health service structure there is no market, and hence no pricing mechanism. A possible way around this problem perhaps is to study conditions in countries broadly similar to Britain where markets in health care do operate, and then use the results as proxies for Britain. Otherwise the only remaining way to arrive at any sort of meaningful estimates is to revert to the method usually applied in the public sector, namely, to evaluate outputs by way of input values.

(4) There are always difficult questions of demarcation between sectors in this kind of exercise, e.g. should teaching expenditure for medical care be included in the health or the education account?

(5) Two additional and difficult problems concerned the choice of

the degree of disaggregation of the overall system and, allied to this, the choice of a suitable sector breakdown. These aspects need very careful investigation, not merely from the viewpoint of internal consistency, but also from the viewpoint of operational feasibility. In the last analysis what one wants is a consistent and *workable* breakdown of aggregates. Presumably, to be of any use at the decision-making level the framework would require disaggregation into considerable detail. However, the question which then arises is whether sufficient and adequate data can be assembled to fill in the different theoretical 'boxes' in a way which is relevant to practical policy.

(6) A special problem in the area of health care is the existence of substantial amounts of volunteer (unpaid) staff resources. The presence of these resources presents serious problems of evaluation. One possible solution is to use as a proxy the value of the labour one might have hired in the market to do the jobs now undertaken by volunteer labour. However, the problem is then one of over-valuation, since if one does not employ paid labour it is presumably because the latter's price is too high.

In the framework of the debate on the social accounting of health, there was also a brief exchange of views on the question whether the percentage share of health in the GNP (and, allied to this, international comparisons of this share) can be viewed as a useful guide to the formulation of practical policy. One participant made a clear distinction between the use of the measure in what he termed *technocratic* terms on the one hand and *political* terms on the other. The discussion was confined almost entirely to the first interpretation. The view seemed to prevail that in a technocratic (economic) sense the measure is largely irrelevant as a guide to practical policy. The measure conveys nothing about the underlying issues governing the process of resource allocation. The real issues are about marginal adjustments in the allocation of resources between different uses, influenced by factors such as opportunity costs, diverging income elasticities for various types of goods, etc. The percentage share of health in the GNP does not enter directly into these considerations. Hence its use by policy-makers, both at the national level and in comparison to other countries, should preferably be discouraged whenever possible.

The potential use of the measure in its second sense, viz. as a weapon of political and bargaining strategy, was mentioned on a number of occasions but not explored in detail at the conference.

Cost-Benefit Analysis

One concrete way in which economic analysis can contribute toward improving the efficiency of resource allocation in medical care (and hence contribute toward the saving of human life and the reduction of suffering) is by focussing attention on the costs and benefits of individual expenditure programmes. This approach can take on a variety of forms, e.g. studies in terms of total or incremental costs and benefits, *ex post facto* or predictive studies, and so forth. There is little doubt that appreciable progress has been made in these various directions in recent years. Yet, despite this progress it is clear that some of the remaining problems regarding programme appraisal in health care, particularly the evaluation of certain benefits (and, indeed, costs) remain formidable. Even in cases involving features making for relative ease of programme assessment, such as in the case of screening for pulmonary TB, some problems remain virtually insoluble.

The central problems underlying exercises of (economic) programme assessment in medical care (as, indeed, in other areas) are mainly twofold, namely, first to identify and isolate the precise effects of a particular investment or expenditure programme, and second to evaluate these effects. Several participants made reference to some of the difficulties encountered in trying to find solutions to these problems.

With regard to the first aspect (identification of effects), perhaps the greatest obstacle facing the economist at present is his frequent and at times acute lack of medical knowledge about the natural history of various diseases and the effects of treatment on the course of these diseases. A second difficulty concerns the fact that, in medical care perhaps more than in other areas, a part of the benefits resulting from a particular investment programme may be predominantly 'non-economic' in character but nonetheless still highly relevant for arriving at decisions about practical policy. The treatment of old people is a case in point which was mentioned by one participant in this context. The provision of health care for old people produces as a rule no direct 'economic' benefits (in terms of increase of output per head or such like) but this does in no way entitle the decision-maker to rule out such provision. In other words, the presumption cannot be that in health care the relevant policy magnitudes are the 'economic' benefits to which any other benefits (biological, social) can somehow be added in a loose and incidental fashion. In the last analysis what is required is a weighting system to judge the various benefits and also a common yardstick to bring these benefits together into a common valuation measure. A one-sided concentration on 'economic' benefits alone, it was said, could carry the danger that in time the medical profession would simply tend to disregard the work of the economist.

In connection with the debate on the identification of effects, reference was also made by some participants to the existence of *ethical* constraints which often impede the proper medical and economic assessment of particular programmes. Typical examples in point here are the ethical limitations often imposed on the conduct of controlled trials on samples of cases to determine the effectiveness of a particular treatment. In the case of lung cancer, for example, it would surely be considered unethical to operate only on a certain proportion of a sample of patients and not on the rest in order to evaluate the effectiveness of the treatment. Similarly, in the case of cancer of the cervix it would almost certainly be regarded as unethical to apply the smear test to only one-half of a group of women and not to the other half in order to gain more information about the efficacy of the test. Against this, one conferee noted that, on the other hand, in some cases it might also be considered unethical *not* to carry out a particular trial.

There was recognition that ethical limitations do frequently have a constraining influence on the scope of programme assessment in health care. The fact must be faced, it was said, that somewhere and at some time in the system, judgements about ethics are being made which cannot be ignored by researchers. Moreover, these judgements are not static; they are likely to change in the course of time. A question which might be asked is: who has the right to make these judgements and when are they made?

One conferee expressed the view that at some time it might be a useful exercise for economists to study the economic implications of ethics in medicine. Another participant thought that by channelling more resources into research now it might be possible to minimise the need for ethical questions to arise in the future. Ethical questions

L

and the frequent consequent wastefulness of medical resources stem to a large extent from ignorance about illness, which would be reduced by research.

With regard to the second basic aspect (evaluation of benefits), a crucial difficulty is that in a non-market situation like that prevailing in Britain today, 'observed prices' are extremely questionable devices to signal opportunity costs to the assessors of a programme. Moreover, there are frequently difficult problems concerning the whole rationale of some benefits. Take for example the specific case of time-saving benefits. For consistency's sake these benefits must be included, but how should they be valued? Is one minute saved twenty times equal to twenty minutes saved at one time? Another important aspect is that presumably only a part of the benefits and costs in medical care will be measurable with any sort of degree of accuracy at all. There are many values in the health care field that will not yield to quantification in the sense of precise and objective measurement. How, it was said, is one, for example, to value precisely human life or the physical and psychic benefits resulting from reduced suffering and anxiety, both to the individual himself and to the community in general.

Finally, there is also the problem of the form in which the results of programme appraisal exercises are presented. Two participants specifically questioned the practice often followed of presenting results in terms of exact figures. There are serious problems attached to the use of exact figures. In most cases, it was argued, it would be more appropriate and true to fact to state the results in terms of *ranges*, or to utilise a more properly statistical (probability) approach. In some cases the decision-makers may not even require precise estimations at all and may be satisfied with a simple classification (viz. 'shopping-list') of the various benefits.

PROBLEMS OF POLICY

Allocation and Distribution of Medical Resources
Since its inception in 1948, the NHS has tried to attain two main objectives: first, a more efficient use of the country's medical resources, and second, a more equitable distribution of health care services between different regions. The four days of discussion at the conference revealed at various points that some participants had

serious doubts about the capability of the present health service structure to achieve these objectives.

Efficient allocation. The removal of the market mechanism means that an alternative method must be utilised to allocate resources in the health service structure. In practice, this means essentially replacing the market place by a system of coherent and interdependent decisions by administrators according to what they conceive to be in the best interest of the community. Several participants had reservations about the validity of this model for the actual world situation prevailing at present in the NHS. The point was made that in many ways the methods of delivery of health care in the traditional services nowadays are still ruled by *tradition* rather than by any rational analysis of particular conditions. This was confronted by one participant with the situation in industry, where economics has frequently broken down tradition and in consequence where rational assessments in allocation (e.g. in terms of substituting cheap for expensive medical resources) is easier to achieve. Also, the view that administrators are governed by consumers' interests when taking decisions about allocation is true only when the system operates perfectly. In practice, however, administrators seem at times to consider consumers' interests less than, for example, the producers' convenience (or their own convenience), and decisions are taken primarily on the ground of expediency. Another point which was stressed by some conferees is that, by tradition, administrators are frequently inclined not to make full use of the powers which are vested in them by virtue of the law. This reluctance is not due merely to a natural and understandable sense of caution, but frequently is simply due to the fact that the central decision-makers do not have adequate quantitative information available on which to base rational judgements. An additional and important factor restricting the administrators' scope of action lies in the present organisation of the health service structure itself, which allows almost complete freedom to the medical profession in the way spending is initiated and the delivery of health care is organised.

There was some concern over this alleged reluctance on the part of the central decision-makers in the NHS to exercise fully the power which is assigned to them within the NHS structure. One participant in particular noted that if this is in fact the case, then this means that, with the absence of markets, we are in danger of being left in the worst of all possible worlds with no coherent and functionally inter-dependent body of decisions for allocating resources at all. Under these conditions the question arises whether there has been any change at all in the misallocations of resources since the inception of the NHS in 1948—misallocations which were one of the chief justifica-tions for the birth of the NHS in the first place.

In reply to this another participant warned against exaggerating the alleged impotence of the central decision-makers in the NHS to control and direct the operation of the system. His own impression was that in fact they had very considerable power to influence the way in which medical care is delivered in Britain. Referring mainly to the delivery of health care by GPs, he mentioned in support of his point the power of the Department of Health and Social Security to influence such features as the employment of ancillary workers by GPs and the potential movement of GPs into group practice.

Distributional equality. With respect to this objective, much of the debate revolved around some of the conclusions reached in one of the conference papers (M. H. Cooper and A. J. Culyer, p. 52) suggesting substantial failure on the part of the NHS to achieve (absolute) equality in the distribution of health care services between different regions. The evidence assembled in that paper suggested clearly that marked disparities in the geographic distribution of health care services in Britain still exist, despite conscious efforts on the part of the central decision-makers to even out these disparities in the course of time. Indeed, in some cases the indications are even of a worsening of the situation in recent years. Some participants charac-terised this development as a disturbing (indeed alarming) state of affairs in a system which has been in operation for over twenty years now and of which one of the explicit aims has been to reduce the degree of disparity in the provision of medical care between different regions.

One conferee questioned the whole rationale of attempting to attain a more equal distribution of medical care services between regions. The distribution of potentially available services is irrelevant, he maintained. What we want is not a more equitable distribution of ineffective services, but *effective therapy*, as measured by some ap-propriate index of health. In this sense it may well be that the distribution of available services *should* be unequal between different regions. His own impression was that in this amended sense the performance of the NHS showed up in a rather favourable light. This view was indirectly supported by another member, who stated that health services should, after all, be provided where people are ill and in need of these services, and not where theoretical measures suggest they should be provided.

Another participant, while not disputing the existence of absolute inequalities in the distribution of health care services between regions, drew attention to the need for a *relative* assessment of these inequalities, i.e. an assessment in terms of an appropriate scale of comparison. In the absence of such a scale of reference, he maintained there is really no way to judge the magnitude and seriousness of any remaining inequalities. We should consider changes over time. Do we know, for example, whether in the absence of the NHS the degree of inequality would not have been far worse than at present? Another possibility is to make international comparisons. Here the evidence suggests that abroad the inequalities are often worse than in Britain, which seems to be well on the way toward equality. In the U.S.A., for example, the disparities are far greater than in the U.K.

There was agreement that, without appropriate terms of comparison, one cannot say whether the remaining inequalities in Britain are great or small, serious or harmless or good or bad. All that can be said with confidence is that at present there is no absolute geographic equality in health care provision. Comparisons over time, it was argued, are clearly desirable, since they might demonstrate at least whether we have been moving in the 'right' direction. However, such comparisons are frequently difficult to perform, on account of the absence of adequate quantitative information for earlier periods.

Two participants specifically doubted the usefulness of international comparisons. A comparison between the U.S.A. and the U.K., they argued, would say nothing about the merits or demerits of the NHS in achieving a greater measure of geographic equality in the availability of health care. Different countries have different objectives and different scales of preferences. Geographic equality is an explicit aim of the NHS, whereas it is not an objective of the United States system of health care provision. In the latter, the distribution of health care services is largely according to the patients' purchasing power.

Several conferees made references to some of the factors which might account for the apparent persistence of disparities in the geographic distribution of health care provision in Britain. Among the factors mentioned the following were the most prominent:

(a) the 'inheritance' by the NHS of gross inequalities which existed before its inception. (Several conferees stressed in this context especially the uneven distribution of capital resources between regions at the start of the NHS, although it was recognised that in the absence of pertinent data it is difficult to supply detailed and systematic evidence on this point);

(b) the existence of differences in the incidence and prevalence of illness in different parts of the country;

(c) the existence of difference in the efficiency of resource utilisation in different regions;

(d) the existence of differences in the standard of general amenities offered to the medical profession in different regions, in the first place, of course, between London and other areas; and

(e) the existence and emergence of so-called 'centres of excellence' which have an implicit tendency to create their own demand and attraction for medical resources, and hence enhance an existing trend toward inequality.

There was also mention, but almost no discussion, of the problems surrounding the nature and quality of the indices that have been currently employed to measure geographic inequality in health care provision (to provide some guidance for future regional resource allocation). There seemed to be general agreement that the indices available at present are in many ways limited and dubious. Some participants deplored the absence of particular types of measures, e.g. a measure reflecting the geographic distribution of the *capital stock* in health care services between regions. A number of conferees made suggestions concerning the possible construction of new indices to increase the number of available measures to serve as guideposts for the allocation of resources between different parts of the country. Among the suggestions made were proposals involving such criteria as unmet need, demographic factors (e.g. age/sex structure) and environmental dimensions (e.g. the level of industrialisation in different regions).

The Problem of Incentives

The existence of inefficiencies and other shortcomings in the health service, as at present functioning, raised a number of important questions. One of these concerned the possible establishment of appropriate incentive (or, conversely, perhaps sanction) mechanisms to improve the performance of the system. Several lines of thought developed on this topic in the course of the discussion and the following statements provide a brief summary of some of the ideas and questions which were raised in this context.

(1) The fundamental problem in the establishment of an incentive mechanism concerns the question of objectives. What is the purpose of a projected incentive scheme? Is it, for example, designed to raise the (economic) efficiency of particular individuals or groups of individuals, in the health service structure? Is it meant to improve first and foremost the quality of care at particular levels in the health care system? Or is it perhaps aiming to improve primarily the process of decision-making by individual managers of groups of managers, at particular points in the health service? Clearly, the list could easily be lengthened but there is little benefit in enumerating further objectives. The fact is that there are many conceivable targets for potential incentive mechanisms, and any attempt at devising such mechanisms must begin by specifying the objectives to be achieved. In doing so, one point must be kept in mind: the possibility that different objectives may come into conflict with each other. For example, the promotion of economic efficiency in resource allocation by a particular incentive mechanism may predispose the system to operate against particular types of cases—a fact which may be inconsistent with the objective of equality of treatment in the health care system.

(2) A second question relates to the form which the incentives should assume, concerning above all, of course, whether they should be monetary or non-monetary. Some participants warned against over-emphasising the importance of monetary incentives. There is in practice no simple answer in regard to the factors governing personal motivation, and in this sense what might prove effective in one case may well fail in another. In some cases non-monetary incentives, say, in terms of greater personal clinical freedom or the chance to acquire new items of equipment to create better and more efficient

working environments, may well prove far more effective in influencing personal behaviour than money.

(3) A third problem concerns the choice of individuals to whom the incentive scheme should be directed. Theoretically, a whole range of individuals might be offered incentives. In most cases the immediate beneficiaries of incentives will be identical with the individuals whose performance is to be improved, but this need not necessarily be so in every case. The possibility of indirect incentives via third parties must be kept in mind. Moreover, as one participant remarked, one need not think merely in terms of incentives to individuals. There is also the possibility of *team* incentives (team bonuses). In this respect, and perhaps also with regard to the whole question of incentives generally, we might be able to benefit from reviewing the experience of other countries, not least perhaps that of Eastern European countries in relation to the management of their nationalised industries.

(4) A fourth aspect concerns the administration and organisation of a prospective incentive mechanism. Should the administration and organisation of such a scheme be centralised or should it preferably be decentralised? And, if the latter, to what extent and in what way? Some groups in the health service structure might well be left to organise and run their own incentive schemes without encroachment on the part of the central managers. One participant mentioned as a specific example in this context, the possibility of GPs' setting up their own incentive schemes without necessarily letting information about them be passed on to the centre of the health service management. The organisation and administration of an incentive mechanism will in the last instance presumably vary, depending on its targets, form, etc. It is difficult to give any *a priori* answers concerning this subject.

(5) Finally, there is the important problem of the quantitative evaluation of an incentive scheme. Clearly, any practical assessment of a particular mechanism presupposes the existence of a set of meaningful and measurable magnitudes to quantify the basis and performance of a scheme. Without such measures, even the best-conceived incentive scheme will remain largely irrelevant for practical purposes.

This question of proper quantification can present some difficult problems, as was clearly highlighted on two particular occasions in the discussion. The participants were debating the general question of incentives, and in this context turned their attention briefly to the consideration of two specific proposals which aimed to enhance the (economic) efficiency of treatment by consultants by providing the latter with more information about the cost of treatment. The first proposal referred specifically to the possibility of regularly 'feeding back' to specialists certain figures about treatment costs, e.g. figures about cost per case. This suggestion drew some critical comments on the numerous ambiguities surrounding the concept of cost in practice. One such ambiguity concerns the distinction of cost in an accounting sense and in a real resource-transfer sense (opportunity cost). Another is that, in practice, cost per case will mean essentially *average* cost per case which, from the point of view of promoting greater economic efficiency, cannot be regarded as truly useful. What one really wants are estimates about *marginal* costs of treatment, i.e. costs which vary directly with the treatment of different individuals by consultants. However, in practice it is highly questionable whether meaningful marginal cost figures can be arrived at.

The second proposal referred to the possibility of enhancing the cost-awareness of specialists by asking the latter to provide *pro forma* bills for the treatment of different individuals, i.e. bills which would provide information about the various costs of treatment without involving the patient in any actual payment. Several participants were quick to point out some of the more obvious shortcomings inherent in such a procedure. How, for example, it was said, would specialists cost their own time in such an exercise? Also, there would presumably need to be some measure of the quality of treatment included in such estimates. One participant held strong reservations about the practicability of this suggestion in the British context. In the absence of a proper market system for health care, the derived figures would be in danger of being largely irrelevant (indeed, mis-leading). Against this, other conferees thought that the figures could be made at least partly meaningful and hence useful for practical policy, especially if at some stage they could be coupled with some appropriate measure of output. At present, it was said, diseases are treated largely irrespective of costs. Hence there would seem to be a strong case for at least reducing the wasteful use of resources wherever possible. In this sense, it follows that any scheme which promises to lead to greater efficiency in resource use should be welcomed in principle.

CONCLUDING REMARKS

The economic appraisal of medical care is a comparatively new development in the field of economics. The growing interest expressed by economists in this area in recent years has been stimulated by a number of distinctive features, e.g. by the increasing importance of medical care in terms of the use of national resources, the importance of health care as a source of human capital and hence as a potential element of economic growth, and also by the increasingly urgent need to devise alternative criteria and yardsticks to the price mechanism for decision-making in a non-market system for medical care.

Much of the work done so far in the field of health economics has stemmed from a preoccupation with specific problems of practical policy. The accumulation of knowledge achieved so far is impressive. Nevertheless, as the discussion at the conference clearly revealed, much of this knowledge is still fragmented and unrelated and further research in this area is badly needed. The general debate at the conference was useful in eliciting the participants' views on where the more immediate research needs might lie and on how future research might best be organised. It should be stressed, however, that no conscious effort was made on the part of the participants to formulate a systematic agenda for research nor to analyse in depth any possible framework of organisation for this research. A majority of conferees seemed to be in favour of a multi-disciplinary approach to the organisation of research. Several participants underlined the value of particular research problems being tackled by groups of experts from different disciplines, e.g. by medical practitioners, economists, health service administrators and statisticians. One participant made a strong plea for the inclusion in such groups not only of experts with a theoretical interest, but also of members more directly concerned with the translation of research results into practical policy.

The following list indicates some of the topics which were mentioned by the participants as possible targets for early investigation:

(a) the analysis and construction of various health indicators (indices of health);

(b) incentives to more efficient resource use in hospitals and by GPs and consultants;

(c) the problem of institutional versus community care with regard to particular sections of the population, e.g. the aged, the disabled and the mentally ill;

(d) the relation between 'need' and 'demand' for medical care, as compared with other goods;

(e) study and evaluation of the economic consequences of group practices and the new contract for GPs in Britain; and

(f) cost-benefit analyses of industrial diseases.

LIST OF PARTICIPANTS

BARR, Dr A.	Oxford Regional Hospital Board, Oxford.
BERESFORD, J. C.	London School of Hygiene and Tropical Medicine, London.
BEVAN, J. M.	Faculty of Social Sciences, University of Kent, Canterbury.
BURBRIDGE, Dr D.	Department of Health and Social Security, London.
CARSTAIRS, Mrs V.	Research and Intelligence Unit, Scottish Home and Health Department, Edinburgh.
COCHRANE, Professor A. L.	Director, Epidemiological Research Unit (South Wales), Medical Research Council, Cardiff.
COHEN, Dr R. H. L.	Deputy Chief Medical Officer, Department of Health and Social Security, London.
COOPER, M. H.	Department of Economics, University of Exeter, Exeter.
CROMBIE, Dr D. L.	Director, General Practice Research Unit, The Royal College of General Practitioners, Birmingham.
CULYER, A. J.	Department of Economics and Related Studies, University of York, York.
CURNOW, Professor R. N.	Department of Applied Statistics, and Director, Nuffield Operational Research (Health Services) Unit, University of Reading, Reading.
DRAPER, Dr P.	Department of Community Medicine, Guy's Hospital Medical School, London.
FORD, Dr Gillian R.	Department of Health and Social Security, London.
GRAY, Dr D. K.	Department of Health and Social Security, London.

HAUSER, Dr M. M.	Institute of Social and Economic Research, University of York, York.
HEASMAN, Dr M. A.	Research and Intelligence Unit, Scottish Home and Health Department, Edinburgh.
JEFFERS, Professor J. R.	Department of Economics, College of Business Administration, and Director, Health Economics Research Center, University of Iowa, Iowa, U.S.A.
LAING, W.	Office of Health Economics, London.
LAVERS, R. J.	Institute of Social and Economic Research, University of York, York
LEES, Professor D. S.	Department of Industrial Economics, University of Nottingham, Nottingham.
LEVITT, M. S.	H.M. Treasury, London.
LEVY, Professor E.	Ministère de la Santé Publique et de la Securité Sociale, Paris, France.
LUCK, G. M.	Institute for Operational Research, Coventry.
MILNE, R. G.	Department of Political Economy, University of Glasgow, Glasgow.
NEWELL, Professor D. J.	Nuffield Department of Industrial Health, University of Newcastle Upon Tyne, Newcastle Upon Tyne,
PIACHAUD, D.	Department of Health and Social Security, London.
POLE, J. D.	Department of Economics, University College of South Wales and Monmouthshire, Cardiff.
RUDOE, W.	Department of Health and Social Security, London.
SALTER, H. C.	Department of Health and Social Security, London.
SHANNON, J. R.	Department of Economics and Related Studies, University of York, York.

SPEK, Dr J. E.   Department of Economics, University of Gothenburg, Gothenburg, Sweden.

SUTCLIFFE, Mrs E. M.   Institute of Social and Economic Research, University of York, York.

WILLIAMS, Professor A. H.   Department of Economics and Related Studies, University of York, York.

WILSON, Dr J. M. G.   Department of Health and Social Security, London.

WISEMAN, Professor J.   Director, Institute of Social and Economic Research, University of York, York.